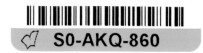
WITHDRAWN

K. *Wayne Smith*
Editor

OCLC 1967-1997:
Thirty Years
of Furthering Access
to the World's Information

OCLC 1967-1997: Thirty Years of Furthering Access to the World's Information has been co-published simultaneously as *Journal of Library Administration*, Volume 25, Numbers 2/3 and 4 1998.

Pre-publication
REVIEWS,
COMMENTARIES,
EVALUATIONS . . .

"**W**ayne Smith has managed the nearly impossible with this book. As he prepares to retire, he has focused not on his accomplishments, but on the contributions this 30-year-old organization has made to the library community. By drawing on authors from the many parts of this varied community, Smith has produced a rich–and poignantly personal, at times–historical account of what is surely one of this century's most important developments in librarianship.

The essays reveal much history, complete with some of the bitter truths and occasional humor about individual episodes of OCLC's development. Throughout, one unarticulated theme becomes dramatically apparent: the leadership Wayne Smith has provided this organization is a story in its own right."

Deanna B. Marcum, PhD
President
Council on Library and Information Resources
Washington, DC

More pre-publication
REVIEWS, COMMENTARIES, EVALUATIONS . . .

"In view of the importance of OCLC to the world of scholarship and learning generally and the library world in particular, this thirty-year review is timely. For those of us who have had direct contact with this remarkable institution (their number must be legion), the book is especially important.

This is no ordinary 'how we did it good' book. The writers of the individual chapters have done an excellent job of assessing the beginnings of OCLC, the changes that have occurred as a result of technological advance, the importance of the revolution in cataloging, and the changes in the way librarians now deliver services to their patrons. The aim of course is to give scholars and the ordinary citizen the services he or she needs when they need it.

Who, in 1968, could have foreseen the changes that this fledgling organization would make, not only in cataloging but also the direct service to readers? The testimonials are appropriate and well written; the authors include some of the profession's most knowledgeable people. They are not limited to the U.S. but include authors around the globe: Asia, Europe, China, Latin America. Among those who particularly interested me were Sharon Rogers and Charlene Hurt's fine piece on 'Electronic Scholarship and Libraries; Or the Medium Became the Message'; Kate Nevins', 'An Ongoing Revolution: Resource Sharing and OCLC'; Christine Deschamps on 'OCLC in Europe'; and of course Wayne Smith's introduction, but especially his conclusion, 'OCLC: Yesterday, Today and Tomorrow.' Smith's essay is an excellent survey of where OCLC has been and where it will be going in the future.

While some persons will read only specific essays, almost all persons will find individual essays of great interest to them. This book is a major contribution to our professional literature as well as to our practice of the profession."

Edward G. Holley
William Rand Kenan, Jr. Professor Emeritus
School of Information and Library Science
The University of North Carolina at Chapel Hill

"**T**his book pulls together in a single source some very interesting historical information regarding OCLC. Perhaps even more important, it depicts the future trajectory of the organization by providing so much interesting detail on the past and present.

The chapter on 'Research at OCLC' was of particular interest to me as I was there at its inception. While no words can adequately capture the excitement that existed as OCLC investigated home delivery via Channel 2000 or created the first interactive book club on Warner Qube two-way cable television, this chapter comes close. It further provides insight into the growth and responsiveness of the organization to the changing needs of OCLC and its constituency.

The book should be of interest to all involved with, or served by, OCLC–and that includes many, many people."

W. David Penniman, PhD
Director, Center for Information Studies
University of Tennessee, Knoxville

"**O**CLC 1967-1997: Thirty Years of Furthering Access to the World's Information *chronicles the remarkable history of a unique and uniquely successful non-profit organization. For those who helped create this extraordinary, now international, institution the book is a walk down memory lane as well as ample vindication of the effort invested. For those who are unfamiliar with OCLC, the work is a lesson in the organizing power of a vision, fueled by member cooperation.

It is entirely fitting that this 30-year retrospective of OCLC should be, itself, a collaborative effort. Taken as a collection, the essays mirror the membership strength of OCLC, the organization. The total is vastly more than the sum of the parts.

Librarians, social and business historians, policy makers, organizational specialists, and all students of the non-profit organization will benefit from the experience, wisdom, and business strategy reflected in these essays."

Ann J. Wolpert, MLS
Director
MIT Libraries
Cambridge, Massachusetts

OCLC 1967-1997:
Thirty Years of Furthering Access
to the World's Information

OCLC 1967-1997: Thirty Years of Furthering Access to the World's Information has been co-published simultaneously as *Journal of Library Administration,* Volume 25, Numbers 2/3 and 4 1998.

The *Journal of Library Administration* Monographs/"Separates"

Planning for Library Services: A Guide to Utilizing Planning Methods for Library Management, edited by Charles R. McClure

Financial Planning for Libraries, edited by Murray S. Martin

Marketing and the Library, edited by Gary T. Ford

Excellence in Library Management, edited by Charlotte Georgi and Robert Bellanti

Archives and Library Administration: Divergent Traditions and Common Concerns, edited by Lawrence J. McCrank

Legal Issues for Library and Information Managers, edited by William Z. Nasri

Pricing and Costs of Monographs and Serials: National and International Issues, edited by Sul H. Lee

Management Issues in the Networking Environment, edited by Edward R. Johnson

Library Management and Technical Services: The Changing Role of Technical Services in Library Organizations, edited by Jennifer Cargill

Computing, Electronic Publishing, and Information Technology: Their Impact on Academic Libraries, edited by Robin N. Downes

Acquisitions, Budgets, and Material Costs: Issues and Approaches, edited by Sul H. Lee

The Impact of Rising Costs of Serials and Monographs on Library Services and Programs, edited by Sul H. Lee

Creativity, Innovation, and Entrepreneurship in Libraries, edited by Donald E. Riggs

Human Resources Management in Libraries, edited by Gisela M. Webb

Managing Public Libraries in the 21st Century, edited by Pat Woodrum

Library Education and Employer Expectations, edited by E. Dale Cluff

Training Issues and Strategies in Libraries, edited by Paul M. Gherman and Frances O. Painter

Library Material Costs and Access to Information, edited by Sul H. Lee

Library Development: A Future Imperative, edited by Dwight F. Burlingame

Personnel Administration in an Automated Environment, edited by Philip E. Leinbach

Strategic Planning in Higher Education: Implementing New Roles for the Academic Library, edited by James F. Williams II

Creative Planning for Library Administration: Leadership for the Future, edited by Kent Hendrickson

Budgets for Acquisitions: Strategies for Serials, Monographs, and Electronic Formats, edited by Sul H. Lee

Managing Technical Services in the 90's, edited by Drew Racine

Library Management in the Information Technology Environment: Issues, Policies, and Practice for Administrators, edited by Brice G. Hobrock

The Management of Library and Information Studies Education, edited by Herman L. Totten

Vendor Evaluation and Acquisition Budgets, edited by Sul H. Lee

Developing Library Staff for the 21st Century, edited by Maureen Sullivan

Collection Assessment and Acquisitions Budgets, edited by Sul H. Lee

Leadership in Academic Libraries: Proceedings of the W. Porter Kellam Conference, The University of Georgia, May 7, 1991, edited by William Gray Potter

Integrating Total Quality Management in a Library Setting, edited by Susan Jurow and Susan B. Barnard

Catalysts for Change: Managing Libraries in the 1990s, edited by Gisela M. von Dran and Jennifer Cargill

The Role and Future of Special Collections in Research Libraries: British and American Perspectives, edited by Sul H. Lee

Declining Acquisitions Budgets: Allocation, Collection Development and Impact Communication, edited by Sul H. Lee

Libraries as User-Centered Organizations: Imperatives for Organizational Change, edited by Meredith A. Butler

Access, Ownership, and Resource Sharing, edited by Sul H. Lee

The Dynamic Library Organizations in a Changing Environment, edited by Joan Giesecke

The Future of Information Services, edited by Virginia Steel and C. Brigid Welch

The Future of Resource Sharing, edited by Shirley K. Baker and Mary E. Jackson

Libraries and Student Assistants: Critical Links, edited by William K. Black

Managing Change in Academic Libraries, edited by Joseph J. Branin

Access, Resource Sharing, and Collection Development, edited by Sul H. Lee

Interlibrary Loan/Document Delivery and Customer Satisfaction: Strategies for Redesigning Services, edited by Pat L. Weaver-Meyers, Wilbur A. Stolt, and Yem S. Fong

Emerging Patterns of Collection Development in Expanding Resource Sharing, Electronic Information, and Network Environment, edited by Sul H. Lee

The Academic Library Director: Reflections on a Position in Transition, edited by Frank D'Andraia

Economics of Digital Information: Collection, Storage and Delivery, edited by Sul H. Lee

Management of Library and Archival Security: From the Outside Looking In, edited by Robert K. O'Neill

OCLC 1967-1997: Thirty Years of Furthering Access to the World's Information, edited by K. Wayne Smith

These books were published simultaneously as special thematic issues of the *Journal of Library Administration* and are available bound separately. Visit Haworth's website at http://www.haworthpressinc.com to search our online catalog for complete tables of contents and ordering information for these and other pubications. Or call 1-800-HAWORTH (outside US/Canada: 607-722-5857), Fax: 1-800-895-0582 (outside US/Canada: 607-771-0012), or e-mail getinfo@haworthpressinc.com

OCLC 1967-1997: Thirty Years of Furthering Access to the World's Information has been co-published simultaneously as *Journal of Library Administration,* Volume 25, Numbers 2/3 and 4 1998.

The development, preparation, and publication of this work has been undertaken with great care. However, the publisher, employees, editors, and agents of The Haworth Press and all imprints of The Haworth Press, Inc., including The Haworth Medical Press and The Pharmaceutical Products Press, are not responsible for any errors contained herein or for consequences that may ensue from use of materials or information contained in this work. Opinions expressed by the author(s) are not necessarily those of The Haworth Press, Inc.

Cover design by Thomas J. Mayshock Jr.

Library of Congress Cataloging-in-Publication Data

OCLC 1967-1997 : thirty years of furthering access to the world's information / K. Wayne Smith, editor.

      p. cm.

      "Co-published simultaneously as Journal of library administration, volume 25, numbers 2/3 and 4, 1998."

      Includes bibliographical references (p.) and index.

      ISBN 0-7890-0536-0 (hardcover : alk. paper). – ISBN 0-7890-0542-5 (pbk. : alk. paper)

      1. OCLC–History. 2. Library information networks–History. 3. Library information networks–United States–History. I. Smith, K. Wayne. II. Journal of library administration.

Z674.82.015016 1998

021.6′5′09–dc21   98-15155

                                                            CIP

OCLC 1967-1997:
Thirty Years of Furthering Access to the World's Information

K. Wayne Smith
Editor

OCLC 1967-1997: Thirty Years of Furthering Access to the World's Information has been co-published simultaneously as *Journal of Library Administration,* Volume 25, Numbers 2/3 and 4 1998.

The Haworth Press, Inc.
New York • London

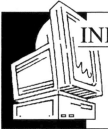

INDEXING & ABSTRACTING

Contributions to this publication are selectively indexed or abstracted in print, electronic, online, or
CD-ROM version(s) of the reference tools and information services listed below. This list is current as
of the copyright date of this publication. See the end
of this section for additional notes.

- *Academic Abstracts/CD-ROM,* EBSCO Publishing Editorial
  Department, P.O. Box 590, Ipswich, MA 01938-0590

- *Academic Search: data base of 2,000 selected academic serials,
  updated monthly,* EBSCO Publishing, 83 Pine Street, Peabody,
  MA 01960

- *AGRICOLA Database,* National Agricultural Library, 10301
  Baltimore Boulevard, Room 002, Beltsville, MD 20705

- *Cambridge Scientific Abstracts, Health & Safety Science
  Abstracts,* 7200 Wisconsin Avenue #601, Bethesda, MD 20814

- *CNPIEC Reference Guide: Chinese National Directory of
  Foreign Periodicals,* P.O. Box 88, Beijing, People's Republic
  of China

- *Current Articles on Library Literature and Services (CALLS),*
  Pakistan Library Association, Quaid-e-Azam Library,
  Bagh-e-Jinnah, Lahore, Pakistan

- *Current Awareness Abstracts,* Association for Information
  Management, Information House, 20-24 Old Street, London
  EC1V 9AP, England

- *Current Index to Journals in Education,* Syracuse University,
  4-194 Center for Science and Technology, Syracuse, NY
  13244-4100

(continued)

- *Educational Administration Abstracts (EAA)*, Sage Publications, Inc., 2455 Teller Road, Newbury Park, CA 91320

- *Higher Education Abstracts*, Claremont Graduate School, 231 East Tenth Street, Claremont, CA 91711

- *IBZ International Bibliography of Periodical Literature*, Zeller Verlag GmbH & Co., P.O.B. 1949, d-49009 Osnabruck, Germany

- *Index to Periodical Articles Related to Law*, University of Texas, 727 East 26th Street, Austin, TX 78705

- *Information Reports & Bibliographies*, Science Associates International, Inc., 6 Hastings Road, Marlboro, NJ 07746-1313

- *Information Science Abstracts*, Plenum Publishing Company, 233 Spring Street, New York, NY 10013-1578

- *Informed Librarian, The*, Infosources Publishing, 140 Norma Road, Teaneck, NJ 07666

- *INSPEC Information Services*, Institution of Electrical Engineers, Michael Faraday House, Six Hills Way, Stevenage, Herts SG1 2AY, England

- *INTERNET ACCESS (& additional networks) Bulletin Board for Libraries ("BUBL") coverage of information resources on INTERNET, JANET, and other networks.*
    - <URL:http://bubl.ac.uk/>
    - The new locations will be found under <URL:http://bubl.ac.uk.link/>.
    - Any existing BUBL users who have problems finding information on the new service should contact the BUBL help line by sending e-mail to <bubl@bubl.ac.uk>.
  The Andersonian Library, Curran Building, 101 St. James Road, Glasgow G4 0NS, Scotland

(continued)

- *Journal of Academic Librarianship: Guide to Professional Literature, The,* Grad School of Library & Information Science/ Simmons College, 300 The Fenway, Boston, MA 02115-5898

- *Konyvtari Figyelo-Library Review,* National Szechenyi Library, Centre for Library and Information Science, H-1827 Budapest, Hungary

- *Library & Information Science Abstracts (LISA),* Bowker-Saur Limited, Maypole House, Maypole Road, East Grinstead, West Sussex RH19 1HH, England

- *Library and Information Science Annual (LISCA),* Libraries Unlimited, P.O. Box 6633, Englewood, CO 80155-6633. Further information is available at www.lu.com/arba

- *Library Literature,* The H.W. Wilson Company, 950 University Avenue, Bronx, NY 10452

- *MasterFILE: updated database from EBSCO Publishing,* 83 Pine Street, Peabody, MA 01960

- *Newsletter of Library and Information Services,* China Sci-Tech Book Review, Library of Academia Sinica, 8 Kexueyuan Nanlu, Zhongguancun, Beijing 100080, People's Republic of China

- *OT BibSys,* American Occupational Therapy Foundation, P.O. Box 31220, Rockville, MD 20824-1220

- *PASCAL, c/o Institute de L'Information Scientifique et Technique,* Cross-disciplinary electronic database covering the fields of science, technology & medicine. Also available on CD-ROM, and can generate customized retrospective searches. For more information: INIST, Customer Desk, 2, allee du Parc de Brabois, F-54514 Vandoeuvre Cedex, France, http//www.inist.fr

- *Public Affairs Information Bulletin (PAIS),* Public Affairs Information Service, Inc., 521 West 43rd Street, New York, NY 10036-4396

- *Referativnyi Zhurnal (Abstracts Journal of the All-Russian Institute of Scientific and Technical Information),* 20 Usievich Street, Moscow 125 219, Russia

- *Trade & Industry Index,* Information Access Company, 362 Lakeside Drive, Foster City, CA 94404

(continued)

SPECIAL BIBLIOGRAPHIC NOTES

related to special journal issues (separates)
and indexing/abstracting

❏ indexing/abstracting services in this list will also cover material in any "separate" that is co-published simultaneously with Haworth's special thematic journal issue or DocuSerial. Indexing/abstracting usually covers material at the article/chapter level.

❏ monographic co-editions are intended for either non-subscribers or libraries which intend to purchase a second copy for their circulating collections.

❏ monographic co-editions are reported to all jobbers/wholesalers/approval plans. The source journal is listed as the "series" to assist the prevention of duplicate purchasing in the same manner utilized for books-in-series.

❏ to facilitate user/access services all indexing/abstracting services are encouraged to utilize the co-indexing entry note indicated at the bottom of the first page of each article/chapter/contribution.

❏ this is intended to assist a library user of any reference tool (whether print, electronic, online, or CD-ROM) to locate the monographic version if the library has purchased this version but not a subscription to the source journal.

❏ individual articles/chapters in any Haworth publication are also available through the Haworth Document Delivery Service (HDDS).

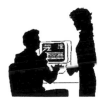

ABOUT THE EDITOR

K. Wayne Smith, PhD, has been President and Chief Executive Officer of OCLC Online Computer Library Center, Inc., Dublin, Ohio, since 1989.

He received the BA in political science from Wake University and the MA and PhD in economics and political science from Princeton University, where he was a Danforth and Woodrow Wilson Fellow. He has also done postgraduate work in economics at the University of Southern California. He received an honorary Doctor of Laws degree from Ohio University in 1992. He was named a Consulting Professor by Tsinghua University in Beijing, China, in 1996, one of only six so honored in the University's 85-year history and the first U.S. citizen.

Between 1964 and his joining OCLC in 1989, he held key posts in higher education, government, and business. In higher education, he has taught at West Point, Princeton, and Wake Forest. In government, he has worked as a "Whiz Kid" in the Pentagon on the staff of Secretary of Defense Robert McNamara and in the White House as Director of Program Analysis for the National Security Council under Dr. Henry Kissinger. In business, he has been Chairman and CEO of World Book Encyclopedia and a Group Managing Partner at Coopers & Lybrand. Dr. Smith is active across a wide spectrum of organizations in higher education, business, government, and international relations. He has served on many for-profit and not-for-profit boards including National City Bank, Scott Fetzer, Wake Forest University, the Mershon Center, and the Institute for International Education. He has written and lectured extensively on national security affairs, systems analysis, information technology, and planning and management. He is co-author with Alain C. Enthoven of the book *How Much Is Enough? Shaping the Defense Program, 1961-1969* (New York: Harper & Row, 1971).

OCLC 1967-1997:
Thirty Years of Furthering Access to the World's Information

CONTENTS

Introduction

In a glass display case under a spotlight in the Smithsonian Institution sits one of the original terminals in the OCLC network. It is part of the National Museum of American History's permanent exhibition entitled "Information Age: People, Information & Technology." In my view, it is not only an important exhibit, but the exhibit title clearly has the key variables in the right sequence, with people first, then information, and then technology.

I believe that it is that same sequence which has helped OCLC to grow and thrive over the past three decades. OCLC has always been technology-based, but long before the technology, there was always the need and the dream–people seeking more and more affordable information.

Technology has changed constantly and dramatically throughout OCLC's history. The Spiras terminal on display at the Smithsonian was manufactured circa 1969 by a company that no longer exists. It was state-of-the-art for nearly a year before OCLC began installing a newer terminal that could be linked to other terminals. The Spiras stayed on the OCLC network, though, for six years before being relegated to obsolescence. When the Smithsonian exhibition first opened in 1990, the Spiras looked quaint. Today, that quaintness has given way to a rugged, pioneering look, almost as if that old CRT terminal belonged in a log cabin. Indeed, with today's chip technology and microprocessors, it is difficult to believe that librarians actually used such a machine as the Spiras to put bibliographic records into a database. But they did!

Thirty years and eons in continuous technological change later, librarians are still putting records into that same database, now called WorldCat–some 38 million records to date. During that same 30 years, WorldCat has also become the most consulted database in higher education. And while the World Wide Web will probably look as quaint to our children's grand-

[Haworth co-indexing entry note]: "Introduction." Smith, K. Wayne. Co-published simultaneously in *Journal of Library Administration* (The Haworth Press, Inc.) Vol. 25, No. 2/3, 1998, pp 1-2; and: *OCLC 1967-1997: Thirty Years of Furthering Access to the World's Information* (ed: K. Wayne Smith) The Haworth Press, Inc., 1998, pp. 1-2. Single or multiple copies of this article are available for a fee from The Haworth Document Delivery Service [1-800-342-9678, 9:00 a.m. - 5:00 p.m. (EST). E-mail address: getinfo@haworthpressinc.com].

children as the Spiras terminal, the information these future generations will be using will have been passed on to them through WorldCat and other innovative databases that today store, organize, and provide access to information. With history's thread now clay tablets and papyrus at one end and fiber optic at the other, this task has become more important and demanding than ever before.

This volume commemorates the 30th anniversary of OCLC's founding as a nonprofit, membership, computer library service and research organization on July 6, 1967. As the 19 articles in this issue show, the OCLC story is fundamentally one of the power of library cooperation for the common good. It is also a story of the age-old dream of people seeking more information and using modern technology to further access and reduce costs. Finally, the story is a tribute to our member libraries, regional networks, international distributors, and most of all, to the thousands of anonymous catalogers and librarians who, keystroke by keystroke, record by record, have created a commons for the world's libraries that has forever altered scholarship and research.

Indeed, OCLC has come a long way in 30 years, but like the Information Age we are part of, we are still at the beginning. As that old visionary and OCLC's founder, Fred Kilgour, once put it: "Like the Wright Brothers at Kitty Hawk, we are only twelve seconds off the ground."

K. Wayne Smith

What WorldCat
(The OCLC Online Union Catalog)
Means to Me

George E. Bishop
Donald O. Case
Patricia L. Hassan
Jeanette C. Smith
Daofu Zhang

INTRODUCTION

August 26, 1996 marked the 25th anniversary of WorldCat (the OCLC Online Union Catalog). As part of a year-long tribute to this remarkable resource, OCLC and the U.S. regional networks sponsored an essay contest in which librarians and library users were invited to write essays of 500 words or less on the topic, "What the OCLC Online Union Catalog Means to Me." A grand prize of $1,000 and four prizes of $500 each were offered.

The contest attracted entries from 340 librarians in 13 countries. These authors used the OCLC bibliographic database in libraries of all types and sizes, including one that measured 12 by 18 feet. The prize-winning essays follow.

[Haworth co-indexing entry note]: "What Worldcat (The OCLC Online Union Catalog) Means to Me." Bishop et al. Co-published simultaneously in *Journal of Library Administration* (The Haworth Press, Inc.) Vol. 25, No. 2/3, 1998, pp. 3-9; and: *OCLC 1967-1997: Thirty Years of Furthering Access to the World's Information* (ed: K. Wayne Smith) The Haworth Press, Inc., 1998, pp. 3-9.

GRAND PRIZE WINNER

by George E. Bishop, Ovid-Elsie Area Schools, Elsie, Michigan

In 1991 our small rural school library was included in an LSCA Grant project giving us our first access to OCLC through Group Access Capability. During the first year of this grant there was significant learning about the Union Catalog. We received excellent support and training from Michigan Library Consortium, our OCLC regional network. We added our holdings through RETROCON, and we did some sampling of the ILL subsystem in order to get our feet wet. After the first year I had learned the power of the OCLC database and was ready to extol its capabilities.

On the first teacher day of the fall of 1992 at the district staff meeting, I announced to over 100 teachers and administrators that our school library would supply *"all* books for any student, teacher, administrator or community member." There was disbelief. Teachers whispered their skepticism during the meeting. Within two weeks, one elementary teacher requested 17 monographs from a bibliography on euthanasia. Our library, using OCLC ILL, supplied ALL the materials she requested. Later I discovered it was a test to see if the library could do what I had promised. We passed the test! The library soon became a credible source for all information. I was not prepared for the domino effect that was ahead.

After gaining the respect of both faculty and students, the library has literally become the center of learning of the school. School improvement teams do extensive research, students use OCLC WorldCat for papers, students get plans for woodshop projects, and graduates now come back to do work for college. Teachers now use our school library to do graduate-level research for college classes they are taking. The attitudes are positive, and our mission of supplying everything for everyone is being achieved. Our OCLC ILL statistics are very high, and so is our level of patron satisfaction.

The most memorable change that has occurred has been in the funding area. Due to the increased visibility and performance of the library and the commitment to providing "everything for everyone," our book budget has been increased from $4,000 to almost $16,000 in only four years. All other budget areas have significantly increased as well. The single factor that started this snowball effect is our access to the OCLC Online Catalog. I now understand that the smaller the library, the more essential it is to have access to the OCLC Online Union Catalog containing the world's recorded knowledge. It is an integral part of the access and learning equation. The OCLC Online Union Catalog has made the single most significant contribution to our small rural school library beyond any book, database, program or person. Through OCLC our library mission has become achievable. Our library and its patrons will never be the same.

PRIZE WINNER

by Donald O. Case, University of Kentucky, Lexington, Kentucky

Herbert George Wells had mixed success as a prophet. In futuristic works written between 1895 and 1938, H. G. Wells correctly predicted, among other developments, the use of airplanes, tanks and atomic weapons in warfare, the growing emancipation of women, the growth of suburbs, and the start of the Second World War in Poland. Of course, Wells forecast many events that have not come to pass, such as the disappearance of warfare, nation states, and large cities.

One of Wells' visions was of a comprehensive World Encyclopedia that he also called a "World Brain."* In his 1938 description of the Encyclopedia, Wells depicted a global compendium of articles, indices and bibliographies that would serve as a central clearinghouse of information for the world's people. The purpose of the Encyclopedia was to capture, synthesize and condense, on a continuing basis, our evolving knowledge of the universe.

In 1971, more than a century after his birth, Wells' World Brain became reality with the initiation of the Ohio College Library Center (later to become the OCLC Online Union Catalog) and the establishment of computer networks to exchange information. By the 1980s the stem of Wells' World Brain was in place, eventually to include documentation of 4,000 years of recorded knowledge.

As a scholar, the utility and importance of the OCLC Online Union Catalog is evident. Twenty-five years ago, when OCLC started, I was a college freshman. At that time a literature search meant leafing through thousands of cards in oaken drawers; my search was only as good as my school's catalog and my own patience.

Now, through the member catalogs of OCLC, I can locate the description and location of almost any publication of potential importance to me. Studying the history of technology, as I do, it is vital that I be able to locate and verify information about older works. I can, for instance, not only locate copies and descriptions of Wells' prophetic books but also film and recorded sound versions of them, as well as editions in hundreds of languages. To be able to do this from my home or office, using an OCLC

---

*Wells, H. G. 1938. *World Brain.* Garden City, NY: Doubleday.

member's system, is a great leap forward for scholarship; and it has been accomplished within the space of one generation of scholars. That's why I think of the Online Union Catalog as my personal version of Wells' Encyclopedia.

Of course, the OCLC Online Union Catalog is not the World Brain of H. G. Wells; OCLC's Catalog does not contain the variety of encyclopedic entries that were described by Wells; but then neither is there the extent of agreement on the nature of "truth" that he imagined possible. The efforts of OCLC are the closest we have yet come to realizing Wells' prophetic vision of a repository for global knowledge.

PRIZE WINNER

by Patricia L. Hassan, Johnson County Library, Shawnee Mission, Kansas

Very proudly I tell you that I have helped to build an international knowledge base–I and many other ordinary catalogers the world over, during the last 25 years. From the largest scholarly institutions to the tiniest public libraries, this grassroots participation in creating the OCLC Online Union Catalog has resulted in an international infrastructure which many ordinary citizens may take for granted–or may be unaware of. But when a medium-size library in America's prairie heartland furnishes materials to the University of Moscow in Russia or the State Library of Berlin, Germany–as a routine function and without fanfare–isn't that a status quo which speaks eloquently of the power of dedicated technology strategy partnered with vision?

The OCLC Online Union Catalog has endowed new power to libraries–and to local library users. It's as if this capability transforms all libraries into "satellites of Alexandria," realizing the rebirth of a long-lost dream of capturing all the knowledge in the world. The ancients who mourned the burning of the Great Library of Alexandria would even recognize many of the works cited in the OCLC Online Union Catalog, since its holdings span 4,000 years of recorded knowledge. The most important part of its name is "Union," because its worth expands and contracts with the gain or loss of any one of the thousands of participating libraries. Rather than being limited to use by scholars, however, the OCLC Online Union Catalog benefits anyone–potentially, anyone at all–who needs information–any information at all, in any format.

Born of necessity, innovation and ingenuity, the OCLC Online Union Catalog has catalyzed a new era of exchange of information among libraries–and a shift in the average person's perception of what is possible in obtaining information, never mind whether that person knows the name of this tool. Its promise–and that fulfillment–fostered new expectations and assumptions and standards about library service. Because the Catalog is such a dynamic, rich resource serving as a foundation for many uses, it has actually become a piece of knowledge in itself. And instead of being "information archives," libraries have become "information access points."

Its impact has been to help launch the global Information Age–in that the scope of information is beyond borders, and cooperation in creating and obtaining that information is a daily, routine affair. We begin to feel that little is beyond our grasp–and to act as if that were true. Wherever technology now takes us and whatever the future holds, the OCLC Online Union Catalog cannot fail to be a cornerstone of the imagination and experience that fuels invention.

Catalogers created this groundbreaking tool, I among them; but as a library user, I am also its legatee.

PRIZE WINNER

by Jeanette C. Smith, New Mexico State University, Las Cruces, New Mexico

Furthering Access to the World's Information.
The Berlin Wall is coming down! An all-encompassing joy filled me on November 9, 1989, as I watched the images on TV. The next day I and my Government Documents staff put up a library display on German reunification. Little did I know that just a few short years later I would be visiting former East Germany to work on a research project. Nor did I realize the instrumental role that OCLC would play during every stage of this project.

Planned as a women's history project, my historiography of sources on a sixteenth century woman, Katharina von Bora, Martin Luther's wife, would have been impossible to complete without the combination of uncensored correspondence, unrestricted travel, and subject access to the world's largest bibliographic database.

I knew that there was more material on Katie von Bora than most people realized, but I was stunned to recover more than 100 catalog records from my FirstSearch subject search on OCLC WorldCat. No amount of time searching individual library electronic or card catalogs could have provided this solid base of information. I had very good luck receiving many materials through OCLC interlibrary loan. In addition, the OCLC Online Union Catalog locations for each record were helpful in planning my travels to see rare book materials unavailable through interlibrary loan.

Upon my return from travels to libraries in the U.S., my database on Katie had grown to more than 200 books and articles, thanks to painstaking tracing of references in books, indices, and bibliographies as far back as the sixteenth century. Despite my efforts, many of these references were still incomplete, and it was time for intensive verification. Again, OCLC came to the rescue as I searched the Online Union Catalog by the traditional author, title, and author/title keys as well as by the PRISM commands. I also used OCLC to verify the language of some titles.

A research trip to Berlin, Lutherstadt Wittenberg, and Leipzig in former East Germany was the highlight of my project. I visited many libraries, interviewed scholars, and walked in Katie's footsteps in many of the towns connected with her life. In Berlin as I looked at the remains of the Berlin Wall, I re-experienced my emotions of 1989. My joy was for mankind, for the breaking down of barriers that divide us. I realized that my project would have remained a dream just a few years earlier. Two factors alone, German reunification and the ability to do a subject search on the OCLC WorldCat, made it a feasible undertaking.

Not only are mankind's physical, political, and economic barriers coming down, but new bridges for international communication and scholarship are being built. Multiply my individual experience by thousands of libraries and millions of researchers, and it is clear that OCLC has truly revolutionized access to the world's information. These are exciting times for us as librarians and as library users. *Danke schoen*, and thank you, OCLC, for helping us to expand our world!

PRIZE WINNER

by Daofu Zhang, Shandong University of Technology, Jinan Shandong, China

Having gone through a journey of 25 years, OCLC has grown up to a brilliant young man in his prime, following his beautiful childhood and smart juvenile years.

OCLC is now taking on a prosperous look. It is a milestone in the field of library information, and also a significant mark of man's entering into the information society. It collects the wisdom of the modern human and has created miracles one after another, shining with radiance and splendor all along.

OCLC has brought happy news to thousands of people. As one of its users, it means a kind of noble enjoyment to me.

OCLC is a gold key which enables me to open easily the gate to all human knowledge and to explore freely the world's treasure-house of civilization.

OCLC is a telescope which helps me realize the old dream of "a thousand-li eye and a tailwind ear" described in classical Chinese novels. While simply sitting at home, OCLC makes it possible for me to look up tens of thousands of introductory passages and whole articles in libraries far away and listen to beautiful music played a long way off.

Using OCLC is faster than riding in a rocket. With it, I am able to travel around the world at the speed of light within a wide span of 4,000 years. OCLC reaches every corner of the world and greatly shortens the distances. It makes the globe magically small and turns a thousand years into an instant by providing the access to any information at the snap of the fingers.

OCLC is to me something like an international pass with which I can "visit" several thousand libraries in more than 100 countries without having to go through the complicated procedures for a passport abroad.

OCLC is a qualified secretary, a good companion and a friend. Whenever I meet with difficult problems in my teaching and research and need to refer to some materials, OCLC is always there to provide me with the best help, making me feel the warmth and encouragement of a relation.

OCLC has become a member of my family. We can no longer do without it. We all love it. I would like to wish the 25-year-old "young man" to be brighter and braver in facing the coming new century!

Users Council:
An Institutionalized Role
for Libraries in OCLC's Governance

Victoria L. Hanawalt

On January 27-29, 1997, fifty-six delegates and four alternates gathered in Columbus, Ohio, for one of three meetings held each year of the OCLC Users Council. The focus of this particular session was "OCLC's Strategic Plan: Partnerships and Beyond." In advance of the meeting delegates had received copies of the latest draft of OCLC's new plan along with a set of questions prepared by the Users Council Executive Committee to help structure the discussion.

The minutes of that meeting record ten specific recommendations crafted by the Council, along with the following statement:

> Comments from delegates emphasized the significance of membership issues, increased international expansion and perspective, cost-effectiveness, and strengthening two-way communication between OCLC and libraries.[1]

This concern for maintaining strong communication between OCLC and its member libraries is hardly a new notion. However, OCLC's willingness to distribute widely a key planning document in draft form and to work with delegate librarians on the substance of that plan are indicative of considerable strengthening of those lines of communication since the creation of the Users Council 20 years ago.

Victoria L. Hanawalt is College Librarian, Reed College, Portland, OR.

[Haworth co-indexing entry note]: "Users Council: An Institutionalized Role for Libraries in OCLC's Governance." Hanawalt, Victoria L. Co-published simultaneously in *Journal of Library Administration* (The Haworth Press, Inc.) Vol. 25, No. 2/3, 1998, pp. 11-18; and. *OCLC 1967-1997: Thirty Years of Furthering Access to the World's Information* (ed: K. Wayne Smith) The Haworth Press, Inc., 1998, pp. 11-18. Single or multiple copies of this article are available for a fee from The Haworth Document Delivery Service [1-800-342-9678, 9:00 a.m. - 5:00 p.m. (EST). E-mail address: getinfo@haworthpressinc.com].

In the late 1970s, libraries outside of Ohio were eager to participate in the setting of future directions for OCLC. In an article published in 1977, Norman Stevens outlined some of the specific concerns of member libraries in those early years of OCLC: response time; system down time; the lack of adequate printed information; a failure to meet announced timetables; and the need to establish firm priorities. He called for some fundamental changes in OCLC governance to help address these concerns.

> Networks and libraries . . . want a real role in the making of the decisions that affect their budgets and their operations . . . One fundamental objective of any restructuring process should be to provide a mechanism for the control of policy decisions that will enable OCLC to be more responsive to the needs of all of its users.[2]

Earlier that year, OCLC had commissioned a study to examine options for an expanded governance structure. The results of that study were detailed in the Arthur D. Little, Inc. report, which recommended "that OCLC establish a governance structure that offers a compromise in character between a 'tightly held, nonprofit corporation' and a 'network cooperative.' "[3]

The Little report recommended the creation of a Users Council, with an aim to formalizing user participation in OCLC. "The purpose of the Users' Council will be to give the networks and other current users of OCLC an institutionalized role, particularly in the making of policy decisions that would directly affect their own operations."[4]

OCLC moved quickly and adopted these recommendations on December 20, 1977. The Users Council held its first meeting less than a year later.

> The Council spent two days talking about priorities and its prospective role. The Council blocked out the following as its top concerns: communication between OCLC operational and management personnel and the individual OCLC users; the implementation of AACR2; the development of OCLC subsystems; quality control within the system; network growth and terminal allocation; and the priorities of OCLC system development . . .[5] Frederick Kilgour, then OCLC Executive Director, spoke at that first meeting about plans for "getting the interlibrary loan mode operational" and for "a new family of terminals, hopefully with a 64K memory . . ."[6]

While many of the issues have changed, a key purpose of Users Council was and is "to reflect and articulate the various interests of General Members" (Code of Regulations, Article V, Section A). But the role of the

Council is not limited to encouraging communication to and from the membership and representing member concerns to OCLC.

Council bylaws mandate a role for Users Council making it much more than a kind of institutionalized focus group. The bylaws state that the Council shall:

A. Encourage and facilitate any OCLC operations, plans, or cooperative efforts that benefit the General Members.
B. Represent the interests and concerns of the Users Council members and their General Member constituents.
C. Expedite the flow of information between the General Members and OCLC.
D. Elect six (6) Trustees of the OCLC Board of Trustees.
E. Approve or reject without modification amendments to the Articles of Incorporation and the Code of Regulations as presented by the Board of Trustees.
F. Engage in other related matters serving the General Members.

It is the mandate to elect from the Council six members of the OCLC Board of Trustees (two members elected every other year to serve six-year terms) that defines Users Council as a significant and continuous component of OCLC's governance structure.

The OCLC Board is composed of fourteen elected members, in addition to the President and Chief Executive Officer. These fourteen include eight trustees elected by the Board itself and the six trustees elected by Users Council. Trustees elected by the Board serve four-year terms. Three of these eight individuals must be members of the library profession. Trustees elected by Users Council serve six-year terms and must themselves be Users Council delegates at the time of their election. Thus the composition of the Board is designed to insure that a majority of members have close ties to libraries and the library profession. Furthermore, any changes to OCLC's Articles of Incorporation and Code of Regulations must be approved by Users Council.

USERS COUNCIL ORGANIZATION

The internal organization of the Council and the structure of its meetings are designed both to support the enhancement of communication with OCLC and to foster the development of delegates as potential trustees. Newly-elected Council members are encouraged to become acquainted with their fellow delegates and familiar with the culture of the organization. They are assigned mentors from among more senior delegates who advise them on options for taking leadership roles in Council.

Four committees–the Bylaws, Election Certification, Finance, and Nominating Committees–provide delegates the opportunity to do focused work in support of the Council.

Finance Committee members review the Users Council budget before its presentation at the spring meeting, when the Council as a whole votes on the budget for the coming year. Although members of the Finance Committee are charged "to advise on, and react to, economic and financial issues and concerns as they relate to OCLC and its members," the fiduciary responsibility for OCLC clearly rests with the OCLC Board of Trustees.

The Nominating Committee, which includes a delegate from every network, develops a slate of candidates for the Council's Executive Committee elections and for the biannual elections of OCLC Trustees. The five-member Executive Committee (a president, vice-president/president elect, and three delegates at large) works with the OCLC Program Manager and OCLC leadership to craft a general thematic focus for the year and to develop agendas for the three Council meetings.

All Council meetings take place in Columbus. With the recent completion of OCLC's Smith Building, delegates and OCLC staff have enjoyed much improved facilities for presentation and discussion. The proximity to OCLC offices encourages attendance by dozens of OCLC staff who might not otherwise be able to participate in and benefit from Council deliberations.

In addition to the standing committee structure, the Executive Committee often appoints a task force or ad hoc committee to focus on an issue in need of special attention. Some of these groups have addressed external membership issues, and others have focused on issues related to the internal functioning of the Council.

In 1992/93, the Future Use of the Online Union Catalog (OLUC) Task Force issued a report addressing actions which affect the content, quality, and use of WorldCat, the OCLC Online Union Catalog. In 1993/94, the Task Force on the Code of Responsible Use drafted a major revision of that document, now titled *The OCLC Online Union Catalog: Principles of Cooperation.* The changes in the title and language of this document, which was circulated widely before adoption, emphasize the mutual responsibilities of OCLC, networks and other partners, and member libraries in maintaining WorldCat. In 1995/96, the Task Force on Original Cataloging Credits examined and determined that no major changes are needed in the current credits structure.

Most recently, in 1996/97, an Ad Hoc Committee to Review Nomination and Election Procedures drafted changes in the timeline and procedures for nominating and electing Trustees and officers of the Council. These changes, which were approved at the spring meeting and which will be in effect in the coming year, should strengthen Council's ability to develop strong slates of candidates for both groups.

AN ARENA FOR CONSULTATION AND ADVICE– USERS COUNCIL AS A FOCUS GROUP

The Council does not limit itself to debating the fine points of policy statements or generalities about the future direction of libraries. Council initiatives can have a direct and significant impact on product development timetables and customization of services. For example, the profession had long debated the advisability of offering centralized accounting and invoicing for interlibrary loan (ILL) fees. The issues were not technical limitations. Rather, the arguments against such a service reflected professional concerns that an ILL accounting service would encourage the charging of fees. It was a resolution from Users Council supporting the development and marketing of this optional service that resulted in OCLC's current ILL fee management system (IFM).

To help provide an additional framework for Council deliberations, each delegate serves on one of four interest groups: Communications & Access; Reference Services/Electronic Publishing; Resource Sharing; and Technical Services. A delegate and a key OCLC staff member serve as co-leaders of each group. Each also includes a member of the current executive committee in its membership. The co-leaders work together to set the agendas for interest group meetings. The executive committee often requests that the interest groups discuss a topic related to the theme of the meeting from their particular perspectives.

At other times delegates meet in groups based on the individual member's home library affiliation. Delegates can participate in meetings of large academic, medium academic, small academic, public, or special librarians. While it often is valuable to hear about the concerns common to particular types of libraries, it should be noted that Council delegates serve as representatives of their networks, not of any individual institution. They have a responsibility to reflect the perspectives and concerns of all sizes and types of libraries. As a reflection of that identity, standard protocol for introducing oneself on the floor of Users Council is to give your name and the name of your network before speaking.

AN OPPORTUNITY FOR EDUCATION
AND PROFESSIONAL DEVELOPMENT–
USERS COUNCIL AS FARM CLUB

Certainly OCLC is the recipient of a good deal of advice from Council delegates. However, delegates often express the opinion that the benefits of serving on Council more than compensate for the time and effort required. Some have characterized it as one of their best professional development experiences. Council regularly schedules presentations by OCLC's own experts.

And it is not uncommon for the Executive Committee to select one or two outside speakers to bring another perspective to the topic at hand. Over the course of this past year, the theme of which was "Model Partnership: Building the Electronic Library," delegates heard from non-delegate librarians, trustees, vendors, publishers, and the superintendent of documents in addition to OCLC speakers. Dr. K. Wayne Smith, OCLC President and Chief Executive Officer, regularly addresses the Council and is often an observer at the general sessions. Several members of the Board are always in attendance at Council meetings. Those trustees that have been elected by the Council are among the most regular attendees. In recent years that roster includes Ellen Waite, Bill Potter, Christine Deschamps, and Bill Crowe. The current board chair, Sharon Rogers, also served as member and president of the Council. At some point during the year, the board chair or other board member is likely to be asked to give a presentation for Council. These sessions might provide an update on current board planning or offer perspectives on the work of a trustee and the skills required.

HAVE WE GOT IT RIGHT?

Peter Drucker describes a common hazard for today's organizations, increasingly dependent on information technology.

> Far too many managers think computer specialists know what information they need to do their job and what information they owe to whom. Computer information tends to focus too much on inside information, not the outside sources and customers that count.[7]

Norman Stevens expressed similar concerns twenty years ago.

> . . . it is far too easy for technical developments, determined and directed by permanent staff remote from current library operations,

to become the overriding considerations in the development of programs and services.[8]

In fulfilling its advisory functions as well as selecting many of the trustees charged with decision-making for the organization, Users Council offers an unusual opportunity for delegates not only to represent immediate member interests but also to contribute to long range institutional planning and decision-making. In short, it actively contributes to both the "network cooperative" and the "nonprofit corporation."

WHAT ABOUT THE NEXT 20 YEARS?

Users Council's representation and mode of operation will need periodic attention to insure its continued effectiveness in the decades to come. Internal issues which might merit future examination include consideration of adjustments to the delegate algorithm, the formula by which each network's number of delegates (out of a total of sixty) is determined. Should use of OCLC's reference services merit proportional representation on Council for networks in the same way that contributions to World-Cat now do?

How will the growth of international membership be accommodated in the composition of the Council? The 1996/97 roster included a delegate from Edinburgh (OCLC Europe) and one from Ontario, Canada (ISM). The Code of Regulations and the Council Bylaws specify that "Users Council Membership is equally available for international as for U.S.-based entities and General Members." How can our ways of doing business change to accommodate an international membership? E-mail communications already support speedier and more economical transmission of the daunting number of documents essential to the running of the Council. (Those 10-pound mailed packets are a thing of the past!) Will Council "meet" via teleconference rather than after dinner at the Columbus Marriott? What impact might these changes have on our ability to know our fellow delegates and to judge their potential as future trustees?

In his 1977 article, Norman Stevens summarized some of OCLC's early technical problems and communication difficulties. At the same time he described OCLC (then the Ohio College Library Center) as "one of the most revolutionary forces to affect library service in the United States in the past century."[9]

As the generations of librarians who can remember life before OCLC edge toward retirement, the shared recognition of the power of that revolution may weaken. But one need only look at a graph of OCLC's ever-escalating interlibrary loan activity to be reminded of the impact that OCLC's shared bibliographic database continues to have. And one need only look at this decade's revolutions in electronic resources and reference services to be reminded of the importance of OCLC's mission of providing affordable access to the world's information.

Users Council has proven itself to be a critically important element in OCLC's organizational structure. In fulfilling its combined roles, Users Council has provided a national forum for articulating member library interests to OCLC as well as a training ground for preparing individuals with library expertise to assume the responsibilities of governing the organization.

NOTES

1. OCLC Users Council. 1997. Minutes of the Meeting (January 27-9): 9.

2. Stevens, Norman D. 1977. "Modernizing OCLC's Governance," *Library Journal* (November 1): 2218.

3. Arthur D. Little, Inc. 1978. *A New Governance Structure for OCLC: Principles and Recommendations* (Metuchen, N.J.: Scarecrow Press): 81.

4. Ibid., 82.

5. "OCLC User's [sic] Council Delineates Top Concerns," 1978. *Library Journal* (September 15): 1685.

6. Ibid.

7. Drucker, Peter F. 1995. *Managing in a Time of Great Change* (New York: Truman Talley Books/Dutton): 12.

8. Stevens: 2219.

9. Stevens: 2216.

The Strategic Alliance Between OCLC and Networks: Partnerships That Work

David H. Brunell

INTRODUCTION:
SO WHAT'S SO SIGNIFICANT ABOUT THIS PARTNERSHIP?

Strategic alliances and partnerships are often viewed as competitive necessities for modern, high-tech organizations. Yet researchers have found that the failure rate for such strategic alliances is high. K. R. Harrigan estimates that more than 55 percent of all strategic alliances fail within five years, while the remaining 45 percent last only 3.5 years longer, on average.[1] Bleeke and Ernst found that "the median life span for all alliances is only about seven years, and nearly 80 percent of joint ventures–one of the most common alliance structures–ultimately end in a sale by one of the partners."[2] They point out that strategic alliances among partners of widely different sizes or organizational types are particularly problematic. Larraine Segil, who is rapidly becoming corporate research's answer to Dr. Ruth, also emphasizes the problems inherent in forging long-term, healthy strategic alliances among different types of partners.[3]

All of this makes it that much more amazing that the strategic partnerships between OCLC and the regional library networks have worked so successfully for so long. First developed in the early 1970s, these alliances with regional library networks have been, I would argue, a major factor

David H. Brunell is Executive Director, Bibliographical Center for Research (BCR), Aurora, CO.

[Haworth co-indexing entry note]: "The Strategic Alliance Between OCLC and Networks: Partnerships That Work." Brunell, David H. Co-published simultaneously in *Journal of Library Administration* (The Haworth Press, Inc.) Vol. 25, No. 2/3, 1998, pp. 19-29; and: *OCLC 1967-1997: Thirty Years of Furthering Access to the World's Information* (ed: K. Wayne Smith) The Haworth Press, Inc., 1998, pp. 19-29. Single or multiple copies of this article are available for a fee from The Haworth Document Delivery Service [1-800-342-9678, 9:00 a.m. - 5:00 p.m. (EST). E-mail address: getinfo@haworthpressinc.com].

both in OCLC's rapid development and the prompt adoption of new OCLC services by the library community across the United States. And the partnerships have been a significant factor in the establishment and expansion of high-quality, reliable, diversified service programs in the 16 participating library networks across the country. [The regional library networks that partner with OCLC are listed in Figure 1 along with their World Wide Web addresses.[4]]

As you can see, a number of types of organizations are represented in the regional network partners:

- Government agencies (FEDLINK, NEBASE, ILLINET)
- Private nonprofit organizations (such as AMIGOS, BCR, SOLINET, MLC, MLNC and NELINET)
- Others that are essentially programs of higher education (MINITEX, SUNY).

FIGURE 1. The Library Networks Offering OCLC Services and Their WWW Site Addresses

AMIGOS Bibliographic Council, Inc. [www.amigos.org]

Bibliographical Center for Research, Inc. (BCR) [www.bcr.org]

CAPCON [www.capcon.net]

FEDLINK [lcweb.loc.gov/flicc]

ILLINET OCLC Services [www.library.sos.state.il.us/isl/oclc/oclc.html]

Indiana Cooperative Library Services Authority (INCOLSA) [www.palni.edu/incolsa]

Michigan Library Consortium (MLC) [www.mlc.lib.mi.us]

MINITEX Library Information Network [othello.lib.umn.edu]

Missouri Library Network Corporation (MLNC) [www.mlnc.com]

Nebraska Library Commission (NEBASE)
  [www.nlc.state.ne.us/netserv/nebase/nebserv.html]

NELINET, Inc. [www.nelinet.net]

OHIONET [www.ohionet.org]

PALINET [www.palinet.org]

Southeastern Library Network, Inc. (SOLINET) [www.solinet.net]

SUNY/OCLC Network [sunyoclc.sysadm.suny.edu]

Wisconsin Interlibrary Services (WILS) [www.wils.wisc.edu]

Geographic size, financial resources and breadth of program activities are other key factors that differ dramatically between the regional networks.

Compared with most commercial strategic partnerships, these long-standing relationships among OCLC and the 16 regional networks is incredibly complex. The evolving dynamics of this relationship have embroiled this key group of disparate (and occasionally desperate) library organizations in a continuing dialog as well as an extraordinarily broad range of service activities for more than 20 years.

HOW DID WE GET HERE?

The partnership between OCLC and Regional Networks evolved from mutual needs in the early 1970s (1971-72). At this time the OCLC cataloging system was implemented online in the Ohio academic libraries that had originally formed the OCLC consortia, and a number of libraries outside Ohio began to express an interest in obtaining OCLC services. Both the OCLC Board of Trustees and management wanted to offer services to non-Ohio libraries, since the predicted economies of scale inherent in a cooperative, shared cataloging database would grow in proportion to the number of institutions contributing records to that database.[5]

Fred Kilgour, the founding OCLC director, actually assumed that the OCLC system would be replicated by other regional computer centers across the country.[6] In addition, the OCLC financial situation in the early 1970s was still fairly precarious. It was clear that the OCLC Board was looking for a way to increase revenue so that it could continue the rapid development of the online cataloging system.[7]

In 1970, OCLC reached a cooperative agreement with the Pittsburgh Regional Library Center (PRLC) that allowed nonprofit library members of that network to use OCLC services. The terms of this first network/OCLC strategic alliance were clearly designed to benefit OCLC and its existing members, as well as the libraries in PRLC. In addition to the income derived from selling services to PRLC member libraries, extending service outside Ohio allowed OCLC to use a more favorable interstate telephone rate for all its members and to apply for grants under a national networking initiative.[8] And the member institutions of PRLC received cost-effective offline cataloging products from OCLC. PRLC itself was given an online terminal connection and permission to use it for library services and experimentation, while receiving training, technical support and advice from OCLC staff. An article in the December 4, 1970 issue of the *OCLC Newsletter* predicted that:

>Extension of this prototype linkage between OCLC and PRLC to other regional library systems could ultimately lead to the development of a national information network that would provide greater availability of library resources, improvement of library use and operations and would reduce the rate of [rise in] library per-user costs.[9]

The implementation of full OCLC online cataloging operations in 1971 led to even more requests for service by non-Ohio libraries. The initial partnership with PRLC was considered promising enough to begin negotiations with several other networks: NELINET, FAUL (which eventually evolved into the SUNY/OCLC Network), the Library Catalog of Pennsylvania (which became PALINET), and the Cooperative College Library Center (whose OCLC work was later subsumed by SOLINET).

Kilgour remained adamant that OCLC service outside Ohio would only be provided through partnerships with consortia or networks that had the capacity to support individual libraries and help OCLC expand nationally. At an ARL meeting in May 1972, he was questioned about libraries on the Eastern Seaboard joining OCLC, and replied bluntly:

>First, those organizations aren't joining the OCLC. We will have as members only institutions in Ohio. We can work with other regional systems that are going to be electronic nodes in a national system. It's on this basis we have relationships with the group here in Atlanta, the groups in Pennsylvania and New England, and the Pittsburgh Regional Library Center.[10]

Kilgour's unusual clarity on this matter probably stemmed from the fact that OCLC's legal advisors had decided that the terms of the original OCLC charter made extending membership to individual libraries outside Ohio illegal.[11] Interestingly enough, it wasn't until January 1973 that the OCLC membership finally voted to allow non-Ohio libraries to become members through regional networks.[12]

These early agreements with regional service networks included a proviso that the network would replicate the OCLC system on its own computer as soon as it was practical to do so.[13] For a variety of political, financial and technical reasons this effort to clone OCLC and form a decentralized national network gradually fell apart. By late 1973, OCLC had come to view itself as the central hub of a de facto national library service network rather than one node of a decentralized networking structure. In its January 1974 meeting, the OCLC Board voted to discourage any further efforts to replicate the OCLC system.[14]

OCLC continued, however, to initiate cooperative agreements with regional networks. By 1977, 20 agreements were in place with such organizations, which evolved into the 16 current network partnerships. OCLC's changed policy position regarding the replication of its services by the regional network partners would lead to ongoing controversies with these network partners. But the successful role that the partner networks now play in providing administrative and technical support, training, contracting and billing services for their member libraries had also evolved early, and would provide the basis for OCLC's continuing support of the network strategic alliances.

Of course, the significant revenue derived from the sale of OCLC services to non-Ohio libraries through the regional networks also undoubtedly had an impact on OCLC's continuing use of these strategic partnerships. By FY 1974-75, 62 percent of OCLC's operating budget was covered by revenue from non-Ohio libraries.[15] The same year, libraries in the regional networks accounted for more than two-thirds of the input cataloging on the OCLC system.[16] Between 1975 and 1980, OCLC annual revenue grew by an average of over 33 percent per year, fueled mainly by the tremendous growth of system use in non-Ohio libraries.[17] By 1977, only 13 percent of OCLC revenue came from Ohio libraries, with most of the remaining 87 percent coming through the partner networks.[18]

But the benefits of these strategic alliances were anything but one-sided. A number of the network partners (including, for instance, the AMIGOS Bibliographic Council, SUNY/OCLC Network and SOLINET) were organized for the specific purpose of providing (or replicating) OCLC services for libraries in their regions. And network growth rates paralleled OCLC's extraordinary expansion through the late 1970s and 1980s. This is not surprising, since a network surcharge on the OCLC services used by its members was (and often has remained) a basic revenue source for most of the nongovernmental networks.

In addition, the provision of day-to-day OCLC technical support and training tied the regional networks to their growing community of users more closely than ever before. At BCR, for example, the number of training and customer support staff increased by more than 50 percent in the eighteen months following the signing of the initial contract with OCLC in 1976. And BCR network revenue more than doubled in the same period, although it failed to quite keep up with the burgeoning costs of supporting OCLC services.[19] Staffing at the AMIGOS network also jumped dramatically in 1975-76 to keep pace with the training and support as dozens of new AMIGOS member libraries began using OCLC services.[20] AMIGOS had the forethought to hire a financial manager early in this period, and thus avoided at least some of the cash-flow woes that haunted OCLC and many of the regional networks during this period.

BCR was not alone in experiencing problems in adjusting to the incredible growth rate resulting from new member libraries who wanted OCLC services. But network support of the partnership with OCLC remained enthusiastic, and evidence of this can be seen in a number of areas.

Most of the early LSCA grant projects funded by state library agencies to support the implementation of OCLC services in individual libraries across the country were cosponsored by regional library networks. And networks actively participated in a number of crucial private grant projects, most obviously the famous Kellogg Foundation grants that funded OCLC participation for 350 small libraries.[21]

Almost all of the early training materials for users of the OCLC Cataloging and ILL Systems were developed by the network training staff. The first comprehensive manual on how to use the OCLC system was the so-called PALINET Manual, written by Bob Stewart, the director of PALINET and used by networks and libraries across the country. The OCLC training programs that the networks developed were often expanded into other related areas: cataloging workshops, MARC format instruction, seminars on ILL procedures, etc. But a study of network training activities in 1992-93 found that 46 percent (1,072 classes) out of a total of 2,345 workshops still dealt with OCLC systems use.[22]

The networks were sometimes asked to prepay their OCLC bills to help ease OCLC's early cash-flow problems, and they usually complied.[23] The development of the OCLC dial-up capability was directly funded by the FEDLINK network.

Network directors participated in discussions of OCLC policy decisions through regular meetings with OCLC management, and even had nonvoting representation at OCLC Board of Trustees meetings.[24] Network representation was clear in decisions ranging from the development of record input standards, to the loading of "deferred" MARC records into the OCLC Online Union Catalog. Lower level network staff cooperated with OCLC in enforcing database standards through such arcane organizations as the Inter-Network Quality Control Council.

The critical importance of the OCLC/Network partnership was clearly recognized in the 1977 Arthur D. Little Report that recommended the establishment of the Users Council, "to give the networks and other current users of OCLC an institutionalized role, particularly in the making of policy decisions . . . ."[25] The acceptance of these recommendations by the OCLC Board of Trustees and membership fundamentally changed the governing structure of OCLC, giving the networks a permanent, institutional voice in OCLC policy decisions.

The benefits of the partnership with OCLC also continued to help the development of regional network programs. The networks' ability to offer OCLC services gave them a far more significant role in the provision of day-to-day service to a broader segment of the library community than most had ever had before. In most cases, it also provided a long-term, reliable basis for funding which, in turn, allowed networks to further expand the range of services they were able to offer their member libraries.

So this partnership quickly became a critically important component in the way both OCLC and the participating networks offered their services to the library community. It was a complex symbiotic relationship that benefited all the participating parties. OCLC expanded rapidly, saw exponential growth in revenue, and used this to develop more system components. The regional networks dramatically extended their membership and used the reliable, expanding financial resources to begin offering a greater range of services to their member libraries. The library community used this partnership to rapidly adopt the OCLC cataloging and interlibrary loan systems, develop the MARC databases that became the foundation of their local systems, and also expand their use of related non-OCLC automation systems.

But the very success of this alliance also led to conflict among the partners. Both OCLC and the networks used revenue derived from their partnership to develop new services that were seen by other parties in the alliance as competitive with the spirit, if not the actual terms, of the original partnership.

As the database of MARC records being created as a by-product of cooperative cataloging grew, it became clear that this was a valuable asset. Naturally, controversies arose over the control and ownership of this asset. The regional networks often found themselves in increasingly awkward positions regarding the protection of the rights of their member libraries, OCLC's stated prerogatives, and their own claims on parts of the MARC databases.

Heated discussion between OCLC and the networks on this issue and attempts by OCLC to solve the problem with new contractual terms that the networks felt were less advantageous, led to a series of public hearings in late 1979 and early 1980. Faced with the real possibility of the collapse of the OCLC/Network alliance, both sides backed down.[26] The same issues, however, arose again in 1982 when OCLC moved to copyright the MARC database, and in 1983 when OCLC renewed efforts to revise the terms of the original OCLC/Network contracts.[27]

As in earlier confrontations, when the controversy over these issues threatened to destroy the OCLC/Network partnership, temporary compromises were reached and the operating relationships continued. Ron Diener, Director of OHIONET at that time, summarized the key issues in contention among OCLC and the regional networks:

1. Should or can networks be marketing agents for OCLC? . . .
2. Who owns or controls the OCLC database? . . .
3. How should major policy issues on uses of the online database be decided? . . .
4. Is the contract [between OCLC and the networks] a computer service contract which imposes performance obligations on the supplier of services? . . .
5. Should networks be obligated to enforce the contractual [database] leasing scheme against libraries and monitor their compliance?[28]

HOW ARE WE DOING NOW?

While the troubling issues of database ownership, "third-party use," and the terms of any new network contracts remain unsettled, it appears the Network/OCLC strategic partnerships continue to be strong, productive and mutually beneficial. The stability of the alliances is at least partially the result of the "institutionalization" of these relationships.

Network/OCLC operating procedures have been organized in what is called the Tiered Distribution Program, which is monitored by the complex and arcane processes of the Regional OCLC Network Directors' Advisory Committee (RONDAC). RONDAC includes all the network directors and has been unkindly characterized as a creature with sixteen heads and no backbone. But it offers a reasonably effective forum to discuss issues impacting the OCLC/Network alliances. Potential conflicts between OCLC and network partners have also been more or less controlled through the establishment of the Tiered Distribution Program (TDP). TDP set up several levels of possible network involvement with different OCLC services, along with general guidelines for network service and financial incentives. These efforts have put an institutional structure around the OCLC/Network partnership.

Similarly, the daunting array of task force groups, subcommittees and working regulations that surround the OCLC Users Council act to dampen the impact of contentious issues before they impact the working relationships among OCLC, regional networks and their mutual member libraries.

The willingness of both networks and OCLC to work within this institutional structure has minimized conflict and recognizes the significant role that the organizations play in each others' business. On the other hand, there is some concern that this increasingly elaborate structure will make both OCLC and networks less agile, and less able to accommodate rapid changes in the information marketplace.

In addition, as OCLC has moved successfully into reference database services, there have been ongoing questions about whether the financial incentives will allow the networks to fully recover the cost of providing marketing and support such services, without adding overhead costs that make OCLC products and services noncompetitive in the marketplace. We need to recognize that it is possible for the OCLC network partnerships to become a detriment to the cost-effective delivery of some types of new services in the future.

But both the network partners and OCLC are evolving institutions. As Larraine Segil has pointed out, the long-term partnering needs of organizations change significantly over an organizational life cycle.[29] Seen in this light, OCLC's newer partnerships with publishing firms and other information providers should not be threatening to the regional networks, so long as the existing partnerships with regional networks are allowed to evolve to meet new needs. Similarly, new cooperative ventures between regional networks and information systems developers will not necessarily replace the OCLC alliance in any way.

As Peter Drucker has pointed out, alliances often become more problematic the more successful they are.[30] In a successful strategic partnership the stakes become higher for all the participants, and that has certainly been the case with the alliances between OCLC and the regional networks. These complex partnerships remain vitally important to all the regional networks, to OCLC and to our thousands of member libraries. The plain fact is that none of us can figure out better ways to do the business we need done without our existing partners. That, perhaps, is ultimately the best insurance we can have for the ongoing health of the most productive strategic partnerships in our profession.

NOTES

1. Harrigan, Kathryn Rudie. 1996. *Managing for Joint Venture Success*. Lexington, MA: Lexington Books. *See also* her article entitled "The Role of Intercompany Cooperation in Integrated Strategy: Strategic Alliances and Partnering Arrangements." in H. B. Thorelli (Ed.). 1995. *Advances in Strategic Management: Integral Strategy Concepts and Dynamics* Greenwich, CT: JAI Press: 5-20.

2. Bleeke, Joel and David Ernst. 1995. "Is Your Strategic Alliance Really a Sale?" *Harvard Business Review* (January-February) Reprint Number 95102: 97.

3. Segil, Larraine. 1996. *Intelligent Business Alliances: How to Profit from Today's Most Important Strategic Tool*. NY: Random House. The effectiveness of Segil's procedures are not yet clearly bolstered by other research, although the key factors impacting the success of a strategic partnership that Segil cites seem to be generally accepted, as is her contention that most strategic partnerships fail. Todd Saxton sets forth a useful summary of the research in this area in "The Effects of Partner and Relationship Characteristics on Alliance Outcomes." 1997. *Academy of Management Journal*, Vol. 40, No. 2 (April): 443-61.

4. Note that detailed information on network OCLC services can be found in the various network Web sites. The network Web site addresses are taken from the August 1997 *Network Directory*, a telephone and E-mail directory of OCLC-Affiliated Regional Networks produced in-house by OCLC.

5. These implications were first articulated in the Parker-Kilgour report of 1966. See Kathleen L. Maciuszko. 1984. *OCLC, A Decade of Development, 1967-1977*. Littleton, CO: Libraries Unlimited: 4-7,18-19.

6. Kilgour, Frederick G. 1984. "Initial System Design for the Ohio College Library Center: A Case History." reprinted in *Collected Papers of Frederick G. Kilgour: OCLC Years*. Dublin, OH: OCLC: 106-7. *See also* Marukskin, Albert F. 1980. *OCLC: Its Governance, Financing, and Technology*. NY: Marcel Dekker: 29.

7. Marukskin: 63. For the same reasons, OCLC allowed public libraries within Ohio to join as members at about the same time. See Marukskin: 62.

8. Ibid. 48-49. See also Kilgour, Frederick G. 1985. "Experience and Expectation." in Wilson Luquire (ed.) *Experiences of Library Network Administrators*. NY: The Haworth Press, Inc.: 67-68.

9. *OCLC Newsletter* 1970. (December) No. 20: 1.

10. *Collected Papers of Frederick G. Kilgour*: 243.

11. Their opinion on this was stated clearly and publicly in materials prepared for the March, 1973, OCLC membership meeting. See Maciuszko, 86-87.

12. Ibid.

13. Ibid. 64.

14. Ibid. 114-15.

15. Martin, Susan K. 1976. *Library Networks, 1976-77* White Plains, NY: Knowledge Industry Publications. 33-34.

16. *OCLC Annual Report, 1974-75*. Columbus, OH: OCLC, 1976. 2.

17. Martin: 34. See also Maciuszko, 124, 195.

18. Maciuszko: 195.

19. *BCR Annual Report, FY 1978-79* (Denver, CO: BCR, 1980) 2, 6-7. For further information on the impact of OCLC service–and both the revenue and costs associated with it, see also Brewster, Evelyn, Judith A. Houk, and JoAn Segal. 1991. *The Bibliographical Center for Research, Rocky Mountain Region, Inc.: The First Fifty Years (1935-1985)*. Denver, CO: BCR. 27-28.

20. Kennedy, James H. "The AMIGOS Experience: The Development of a Successful Network." in Luquire, *Op. Cit.*, 17-19.

21. Maciuszko: 163.

22. Brunell, David. 1994. "Training and Educational Programs Offered by the Regional Library Service Networks." in *Educating for Networking–Building New Partnerships: Proceedings of the Joint Meeting of the Library of Congress Network Advisory Committee and the Association of Library and Information Science Education, June 13 15, 1993.* Washington, DC: Library of Congress: 93-98. A short summary of the financial investment associated with these training programs can be found in Brunell, David. 1989. "Developing New Services in Library Networks." in Donald E. Riggs (ed.). 1989. *Creativity, Innovation, and Entrepreneurship in Libraries.* NY: The Haworth Press, Inc.: 113-14.

23. Maciuszko: 142-43.

24. This representation came through the Council of Regions, and later through Council of Computerized Library Networks (CCLN), which was allowed to send up to seven representatives to OCLC Board of Trustees meetings. See Maciuszko: 206-7.

25. Little, Arthur D. 1978. *A New Governance Structure for OCLC: Principles and Recommendations.* Metuchen, NJ: The Scarecrow Press: 82.

26. A good summary of various aspects of this matter can be found in Martin, 35-39.

27. A scholarly (and very diplomatic) discussion of the general issue of network database copyrights can be found in Oakley, Robert L. 1989. "Intellectual Property Issues and Information Networks: A Background Report." in *Intellectual Property Issues in the Library Network Context, Proceedings of the Library of Congress Network Advisory Committee Meeting, March 23-25, 1988.* Washington, DC: Library of Congress: 5-54.

28. Diener, Ron. 1983. "A New OCLC Contract." *OhioNetwork.* (July) Vol. 5, No.7: 1-2.

29. Segil: 50-60.

30. Drucker, Peter. 1993. *Managing for the Future: The 1990s and Beyond.* NY: Truman Talley Books/Plume: 18.

OCLC and Its Advisory Committees

Shirley K. Baker

OCLC, as a membership organization has, since its inception, sought advice from its members, or had advice thrust upon it. Indeed, in the early days of OCLC, user groups sprang up spontaneously. As time passed, OCLC initiated groups to fill needs and gaps. At present, ten advisory committees and many user groups exist.[1] The presence and effect of advisory groups over time was well documented in the beginning of this decade in OCLC's newsletter, with an entire issue focused on the work of these groups.[2]

This article will focus on advisory committees, and specifically the type-of-library committees. Researching this article has brought back memories for the author, of watching, as a library middle manager, the formation of the Research Libraries Advisory Committee (RLAC). The memories are also surprisingly fresh for those others that I was able to reach who were there "at the birth" of committees. It seems that the creation of an advisory committee was a defining moment in the lives of those involved, since it is so vividly remembered many years later. Certainly, there was a critical link between the formation and activities of OCLC advisory committees and developments in the library profession.

OCLC has grown in its nearly three decades from a supplier of catalog cards to a provider of multiple services and a creator of links among libraries. The decisions involved with participating in OCLC have become significantly more complex. While we all thought that our original decision–to give over autonomy in our cataloging to an outside organization (even a membership organization)–was momentous, we now face deci-

---

Shirley K. Baker is Vice Chancellor for Information Technology and Dean of University Libraries, Washington University, St. Louis, MO.

[Haworth co-indexing entry note]: "OCLC and Its Advisory Committees." Baker, Shirley K. Co-published simultaneously in *Journal of Library Administration* (The Haworth Press, Inc.) Vol. 25, No. 2/3, 1998, pp. 31-43; and: *OCLC 1967-1997: Thirty Years of Furthering Access to the World's Information* (ed: K. Wayne Smith) The Haworth Press, Inc., 1998, pp. 31-43. Single or multiple copies of this article are available for a fee from The Haworth Document Delivery Service [1-800-342-9678, 9:00 a.m. - 5:00 p.m. (EST). E-mail address: getinfo@haworthpressinc.com].

sions about OCLC services which are far more weighty. When we 'bought' our cataloging cards from OCLC, we had the actual cards in our possession, even if OCLC did not survive the next year. Now libraries are charging OCLC to create and preserve our primary materials–our journals and our archives, and the decisions to sacrifice autonomy for cost-control, access, and the common good have far-reaching consequences for libraries and for scholarship. The decisions we now make about OCLC products and services have repercussions well beyond the walls of our libraries. In these times, it is imperative that we work collaboratively with OCLC in guiding the decisions of the organization.

The OCLC Board of Trustees has, of course, ultimate responsibility for guiding the organization, and Users Council plays a stronger role than any advisory committee. Nonetheless, the advisory committees bring together the directors of libraries with common interests to guide OCLC. The type-of-library advisory committees helped move OCLC away from hearing primarily from technical services staff or directors with technical services backgrounds, and have strengthened OCLC's movement into reference, collections, and issues beyond the immediate purview of libraries. Finally, serving on the advisory committees is a mind-expanding and educational opportunity for library directors, for whom there are few 'staff development' occasions. Advisory committee members whose terms are up leave the groups with regret and worry about how they will keep themselves quite as well-informed without the OCLC-based opportunities.

RESEARCH LIBRARIES ADVISORY COMMITTEE

The earliest of the type-of-library advisory committees was the Research Libraries Advisory Committee, which grew out of discussions among ARL library directors in the late 1970s. The immediate impetus for the discussions was the expansionist activities of the Research Libraries Group. In an effort to increase membership from the original four (Columbia, Harvard, New York Public and Yale), RLG organizers were approaching library directors and university presidents soliciting participation, and RLG membership was growing fast. Library directors with strong commitment to OCLC felt the need to find ways for OCLC to consolidate and strengthen its services for research libraries.

Research libraries have always been major contributors of original records to the OCLC union catalog, although they have never constituted the majority of OCLC members. Given its extensive membership of all types of libraries, OCLC designed its services to appeal to the broadest group. At the time of RLG's expansion, RLG was designing services intended to enhance collection development and preservation activities, the most pervasive and prestigious research library issues in the late '70s and early '80s.

There was much high drama involved in the competition between OCLC and RLG. Library directors took strong positions on each side. Some friendships between directors were permanently cooled by what was perceived, especially on the OCLC-director side, as excessive pressure to join RLG. This author remembers being at an American Library Association (ALA) conference in Chicago at the time of an open meeting being held at the Palmer House by RLG for libraries interested in joining. Standing chatting in the middle of the Palmer House lobby, for the duration of the meeting, were half a dozen of the major OCLC-adherents, being obvious about their non-attendance at the RLG meeting. Notable among them was the now legendary Hugh Atkinson, then director at the University of Illinois, Urbana Champagne, and one of his young assistants, William Potter, now a member of the OCLC Board of Trustees.

Whatever the motivation for the formation of the Research Libraries Advisory Committee, the committee has served the profession well in its seventeen years of existence. Its first set of members–Harold Billings, Richard Chapin, James Govan, Gustave Harrer, Jay Lucker, Peter Paulson, Donald Simpson, Kenneth Tombs and Joseph Treyz–is a veritable directory of leaders in librarianship. Membership over the years has consistently included upcoming and current leaders. Joanne Harrar and Kaye Gapen brought some gender balance to the group early on, and current membership reflects today's more even gender balance in research library leadership.

The first OCLC-sponsored conference for research library directors was organized in April 1981, where RLAC chair Harold Billings welcomed 58 of his colleagues. They were looking for ways, said Billings, "that research libraries can work together through OCLC's electronic network to fulfill our educational mission in ways that are faster and more economical."[3] After two years of operation, the committee decided to dissolve itself, in favor of an OCLC-appointed group, with geographic distribution of membership and regular terms of service. Thus, RLAC officially dates from 1982.[4] Terms for membership are three years, with one third of the members appointed annually, and the group, until 1996, consisted of 12 members

RLAC has met twice annually since then and sponsors each year a conference for research library directors on a topic of interest to senior management of the profession. The meetings and conferences continue to focus on "committee goals" to identify and define specific programs of research library concerns, to assist OCLC in establishing priorities for implementing these programs, and to facilitate the wider distribution of the products of these programs. Committee meetings regularly include briefings from and discussion with OCLC research staff, allowing an early glimpse into OCLC's work, and affording an opportunity to shape the directions taken.

By 1996, OCLC had significantly expanded its international membership and increased the proportion in the union catalog of records for international materials. It was time to expand the Research Libraries Advisory Committee beyond North America and, in 1996, Jacqueline Dubois of the Bibliothèque de Musée de l'Homme joined the group, bringing membership to 13.

ADVISORY COMMITTEE ON PUBLIC LIBRARIES

Once a pattern for type-of-library advisory committees was established, it was relatively easy for OCLC to create new committees for different types of libraries, with variations suited to the audience. The Advisory Committee on Public Libraries (ACPL) was the second to be formed, in 1984. The birth of ACPL came two years after RLAC had become official. Enough time had passed for the activities of RLAC to be noticed in the profession. Task forces on cataloging microform sets, on document delivery, and preservation had drawn public attention. *Research Libraries in OCLC: A Quarterly,* published from 1981 to 1985, highlighted RLAC activities. By 1984, RLAC had staged three annual conferences for research library directors.

Appointments to ACPL–12 members, appointed for three year terms, with one-third appointed annually–replicated the pattern already established. Membership also focused on directors, with geographic and type and size of library distribution a goal. The goals parallel those of RLAC, but with emphasis on public library issues and links with the Public Library Association. In March 1988, ACPL and OCLC hosted a *Conference on the Future of the Public Library,* attended by more than 50 directors. The Advisory Committee on Public Libraries also identified a creative approach for reaching the largest number of public library directors: ACPL plans a program for the biennial Public Library Association meetings. These programs have been accepted every year for the PLA program and have been well attended. Agenda topics for ACPL, while somewhat paralleling those for the academic library groups, featured, of course, topics reflecting the greater variation in size and type among public libraries.

ADVISORY COMMITTEE ON COLLEGE AND UNIVERSITY LIBRARIES

Two years passed before the next of the type-of-library advisory committees appeared on the scene. The third, Advisory Committee on College and University Libraries (ACCUL), was aimed at the large number of small and medium-sized academic libraries which are members of OCLC. Indeed, while large research libraries represent two percent of the OCLC membership base in 1996, small and medium-sized academic libraries equal 26 percent.

There are 12 members in ACCUL who serve for three-year terms, with one-third appointed each year. The committee provides a channel to share viewpoints and advise OCLC in areas of strategic direction and policy. Nancy Eaton, involved with the formation of ACCUL when she was library director at the University of Vermont, describes the formation of this group as a natural step for a membership organization. Getting grass-roots input from the membership base keeps the organization focused, she stated.[5] ACCUL also strives to encourage cooperative efforts and OCLC services that benefit academic libraries. And, like the other advisory committees, the Committee serves an important function in keeping open lines of communication between OCLC and its members.

The Advisory Committee on College and University Libraries meets twice a year. It does not sponsor programs for the larger community, as do RLAC and ACPL. However, it serves as an important forum for directors of small and mid-sized academic libraries to work together, on issues important to them and with a major provider of their services. Membership in ACCUL is sought-after and prized.

ADVISORY COMMITTEE ON SPECIAL LIBRARIES

The history of the formation of the Advisory Committee on Special Libraries (ACSL) can perhaps be understood as simply rounding out the type-of-library roster. It is likely, however, that the drivers behind its formation were more complex. Special libraries were not initially members of OCLC. Ann Wolpert, who was library director at Arthur D. Little, Inc. at the time, made ADL one of OCLC's first corporate library members. According to Wolpert, the path to membership was a bumpy one.

"The regional networks were afraid that accepting a member from a for-profit organization might cost them their non-profit status. Eventually OCLC and the networks got some guidelines from the Internal Revenue Service and the comfort level improved. Meanwhile the cost justification we had prepared was such a revelation to the network that they incorporated it into their marketing literature."[6]

There were other obstacles to special libraries' participation in OCLC, according to Wolpert. Special libraries feared that showing their holdings on OCLC would allow others to sniff out proprietary research interests. But, the uniqueness of special libraries' holdings, plus their high level of contribution of original records to the union catalog sustained OCLC interest in them, and special libraries were key players in the OCLC community. By 1996, special libraries constituted 22 percent of the OCLC membership, indicating benefit both for the libraries and OCLC.

In early 1987, a Planning Committee for Special Libraries was formed and in December of that year the first meeting of the Advisory Committee on Special Libraries (ACSL) was held. Among the types of libraries included in this committee's purview are corporate, law, medical and theological libraries. ACSL serves to represent to OCLC the concerns of special libraries and to represent OCLC to the special library community and their professional organizations. The Advisory Committee on Special Libraries is smaller than its peer groups, having eight members. But again, as in other advisory committees, one-third of the membership is appointed annually.

COMMON THEMES

All four of the type-of-library advisory groups work to shape OCLC policies and programs, according to the particular needs of each group. It is the author's experience, however, that committee members are well aware that their interests cannot stand in isolation to those of other constituent groups. OCLC's financial and programmatic success depends upon serving the broad community of libraries.

Advisory groups organized by function were created in the late 1980s. These–Access Services, Collections and Technical Services, Reference Services, Resource Sharing–present concerns across libraries. These groups, in particular, reflect the diversity of the larger library community, from community colleges to the Library of Congress (see member list in the appendix). They also brought balance from non-cataloging areas of libraries, as OCLC expanded its services beyond technical services.

In more recent years, OCLC has looked beyond libraries–to the higher education community and the world of research. A five member Higher Education Policy Advisory Committee with international membership provides perspective for OCLC's senior management. And, OCLC retains a small group conversant in computing and communications in its Research Advisory Committee.

The balance of input from libraries of all types, from library directors and from middle managers, from outside the library community, keeps OCLC's programs focused on current needs and helps guide new directions for this membership-based organization.

NOTES

1. OCLC. 1990. "Special Report: Advice and Consent." *OCLC Newsletter* (May/June) No. 185.

2. User Groups and Advisory Committees Directory, www.oclc.org/oclc/man/adcomm/toc.htm; current advisory committees and their members appended to this document.

3. Zubatsky, David S. 1984. *The Research Libraries Advisory Committee to OCLC: An Informal History, 1980-1984. Research Libraries in OCLC: A Quarterly* (Autumn): 8.

4. Ibid. 9.

5. Telephone conversation with the author, June 1997.

6. Electronic mail communication with the author.

APPENDIX
ADVISORY COMMITTEES 1996/97

Access Services Advisory Committee

Sara Aden
Kearney Public Library and Information Center
Bradley Faust
Ball State University Libraries
Jean Hamrick
University of Texas at Austin
Rob Kairis
Kent State University
Deborah Ludwig
Johnson County Community College
Dan Marmion
Western Michigan University
Melanie Myers
Carnegie Mellon University

Mark Parker
Sacramento Public Library
Richard Reeb
University of Wisconsin-Madison
Jeff Rehbach
Middlebury College
Wilson Stahl
University of North Carolina at Charlotte
Susan Turner
World Bank and International Monetary Fund

Advisory Committee on College and University Libraries

Camila Alire
University of Colorado-Denver
Margaret Auer
University of Detroit Mercy
Lynn Chmelir
Linfield College
John Harrison
University of Arkansas, Fayetteville
Michael Kathman
College of St. Benedict/St. John's University

Tom Kirk
Earlham College
Sarah Pritchard
Smith College
Marion Reid
California State University, San Marcos
Robert Seal
Texas Christian University
Jay Starratt
Southern Illinois University at Edwardsville
Jerry Stephens
University of Alabama, Birmingham
Stephen Stoan
Drury College

Advisory Committee on Public Libraries

Don Barlow
Westerville Public Library
John Brooks-Barr
Upper Arlington Public Library
Linda Crowe
BALIS/PLS/SBCLS
Lon Dickerson
Chatham-Effingham-Liberty Regional Library
June Garcia
San Antonio Public Library
William Gordon
Prince George's County Memorial Library System
Carla Hayden
Enoch Pratt Free Library
Laura Isenstein
Public Library of Des Moines
Deborah Jacobs
Corvallis-Benton County Public Library
Jeffrey Krull
Allen County Public Library
Samuel Morrison
Broward County Division of Libraries
Donald Napoli
St. Joseph County Public Library

Advisory Committee on Special Libraries

Felicia Bagby
Northrup-Grumman
Nancy Lemon
Owens Corning
James Lommel
General Electric
Judith Messerle
Boston Medical Library and
Harvard Medical School Library
Eugenie Prime
Hewlett-Packard
Linda Proudfoot
World Bank and International Monetary Fund
Sally Wise
University of Nebraska

Collections and Technical Services Advisory Committee

Pat Anderson
Newport News Public Library System
Shelby Harken
University of North Dakota
Mary Helms
University of Nebraska Medical Center
Ann Hope
University of Georgia
Victor Liu
Washtenaw Community College
Mary Frances Melnik
The Free Library of Philadelphia
Brian Schottlaender
University of California, Los Angeles
Jane Savidge
Victoria and Albert Museum
Pam Rebarcak
Iowa State University
Louise Sevold
Cuyahoga Public Library
Mary MacLeod
Acadia University

Tom Wilson
University of Houston

Higher Education Policy Advisory Committee

Brian Follett
The University of Warwick
Thomas Hearn, Jr.
Wake Forest University
Robert Heterick, Jr.
EDUCOM
Wesley Posvar
University of Pittsburgh
Richard Sisson
The Ohio State University
Sidney Verba
Harvard University

Research Advisory Committee

Edward Emil David
EED, Inc.
Edward Fox
Virginia Polytechnic Institute and State University
Joseph Hardin
National Center for Supercomputing Applications
University of Illinois, Urbana-Champaign
Bernard Hurley
University of California, Berkeley

Reference Services Advisory Committee

Stewart Bodner
The New York Public Library
Karen Campbell
Hamline University
Ulrike Dieterle
University of Wisconsin-Platteville
Roberto Esteves
San Francisco Public Library
Kurt Keeley
American Water Works Association

Dagmar Langeggen
National Office for Research, Documentation and Professional Libraries, Norway
Nicole Martin
Hood College
Linda Moore
Hillsdale College
Virginia Moreland
Agnes Scott College
Penelope O'Connor
Cleveland Public Library
Barbara Rosen
University of New Mexico
Dawn Thistle
College of the Holy Cross

Research Libraries Advisory Committee

Shirley Baker
Washington University
Betty Bengtson
University of Washington
Jacqueline Dubois
Bibliothèque du Musée de l'Homme
Kenneth Frazier
University of Wisconsin-Madison
Ernie Ingles
University of Alberta
David Kohl
University of Cincinnati
Charles Miller
Florida State University
James Neal
Johns Hopkins University
Carla Stoffle
University of Arizona
Winston Tabb
Library of Congress
Merrily Taylor
Brown University
William Walker
New York Public Library

Karin Wittenborg
University of Virginia

Resource Sharing Advisory Committee

Ewa Barczyk
University of Wisconsin-Milwaukee
Tammy Dearie
University of California, San Diego
Paul Drake
Kansas City (Missouri) Public Library
Casandra Fitzherbert
University of Southern Maine
Lone Knakkergaard
Danish Loan Centre
Michael Kreyche
Kent State University
Dorcas MacDonald
Syracuse University
Tim Prather
Austin (Texas) Public Library
Mary Schellhorn
Columbia (Illinois) College
Harold Shaffer
Indiana University
David Whisenant
Northeast Florida Library Information Network
Christopher Wright
Library of Congress

Changing the Tasks of Cataloging

Lee Leighton

When the OCLC online system first began operation in 1971, cataloging was a little known calling outside the library world, and its practitioners freely adapted its principles to fit their particular setting. The adaptations extended to all areas of the field. The catalogers at the Harvard Law Library added an extra half space above and below the collation line on catalog cards "so it would pop out at you." No other reason was ever given. The public catalog at Harvard Law was filed in "logical order" and then alphabetically within the logical sequences. The "logical order" reflected the structure of Anglo-American legal bibliography and was apparent to the law school faculty, but not necessarily to law students. After the catalog was filmed, library staff found it impossible to refile many of the guidecards because there was no apparent order without them.

All library work, like all politics, as Tip O'Neill once said, was local. There were national standards, but they were freely modified to fit the perceived need of each library's clientele. The Library of Congress had been distributing printed cards since the early part of the century which provided full descriptive cataloging including a Library of Congress call number and subject headings, but they could easily be changed. Scalpels and electric erasers were common catalogers' tools that we had trouble explaining to our friends.

There was also a very sharp division of labor among catalog department staff. Catalogers were all professionals, with or without library degrees, who did all the cataloging. In the larger libraries they generally delegated

Lee Leighton is Assistant University Librarian for Technical Services, University of California, Berkeley, CA.

[Haworth co-indexing entry note]: "Changing the Tasks of Cataloging." Leighton, Lee. Co-published simultaneously in *Journal of Library Administration* (The Haworth Press, Inc.) Vol. 25, No. 2/3, 1998, pp. 45-54; and: *OCLC 1967-1997: Thirty Years of Furthering Access to the World's Information* (ed: K. Wayne Smith) The Haworth Press, Inc., 1998, pp. 45-54. Single or multiple copies of this article are available for a fee from The Haworth Document Delivery Service [1-800-342-9678, 9:00 a.m. - 5:00 p.m. (EST). E-mail address: getinfo@haworthpressinc.com].

only preliminary catalog searching and card typing to support staff. The professional catalogers also often researched problematic headings and revised the cards that needed to be retyped. There were variations: some catalogers typed their own cards, some revised the filing in the shelflist and the catalog, and, of course, in smaller libraries the professional catalogers did it all. The actual intellectual work involved in cataloging: identifying a particular bibliographic entity; describing it; providing name and subject access to it; and controlling the form of the headings was the work of the professional catalogers.

When libraries first began automating cataloging through the use of OCLC in the early 1970s, the computer terminal replaced the typewriter, but not much else. While catalogers were getting used to fixed fields and MARC coding, it was still possible to leave the division of labor as it had been and tweak or hammer the cataloging on the printout to fit into your local catalog just as you had done before.

Soon things began to change very quickly, at least in the area of national standards. Cataloging administrators began to ask why the folks were bleeding red ink all over the printouts, and some libraries were starting to close card catalogs constructed by local standards in favor of new ones with machine-produced cards with Library of Congress call numbers, name headings and subjects. Although the switch to the LC classification system had come considerably earlier for most large libraries, and AACR2 was not yet on the horizon, automating the cataloging process in the early 1970s would prove to be the most important change to hit libraries in the next two decades. It also placed professional catalogers in front of a tidal wave of changes. The two most fundamental changes which occurred during this period were:

1. a shift to shared, standardized cataloging, and
2. a new division of labor between professional and copy catalogers

The publication of the *Anglo-American Cataloging Rules,* second edition, in 1978 and its implementation by the American library community in 1981 embodied the shift to commonly held national and international standards. New off-shoot card catalogs appeared in libraries that hadn't had them before. Many older, off-shoot catalogs created when catalog automation first began were turned into computer-output microfiche supplements to card catalogs awaiting retrospective conversion.

The introduction of copy cataloging fundamentally changed the dynamics of the profession. Library support staff were beginning to share some of the same duties as professional librarians. The shift was very slight at first–librarians were naturally reluctant to relinquish part of their responsibilities to staff who were less trained and clearly not equipped to handle all the complications that arise in descriptive and subject cataloging. But the most important change in thinking had occurred: similar kinds of work could be done by different levels of staff. Rather than just searching, typing and filing, library assistants during the 1980s began to operate the computers and handle the Library of Congress copy they provided. After all, the real work had been done by professional librarians in Washington. Processing copy from libraries other than the Library of Congress was still in the hands of the professional catalogers because all those little quirks from other libraries had to be edited out and the local library's added in.

The budget cuts that many libraries experienced in the 1990s brought home the large scale reorganizations, downsizing and scrambling for new ideas that had become commonplace in the business world. Library operations budgets were hit with staff reductions through attrition and early retirement buy-out plans, and technical service operations were often targeted for staff reductions in order to maintain staffing levels in other areas of the library. Catalogers, especially, were victims of their own success in rearranging patterns and kinds of work to maintain production with fewer and less expensive staff. Faster, more powerful desktop computers also moved catalogers through their work more quickly, allowing them instant access to local and national databases. Because catalogers had already faced major changes in their work, many realized that planning for change would become a regular part of their professional work.

It was also a time when the computer revolution in the workplace predicted for the baby boom generation came true. Most librarians and support staff had powerful minicomputers on their desks, and the Internet and local intranets really hooked all of us together for the first time. The new interconnectivity provided a new pathway for information to flow directly from the producer to the consumer; both the reference librarians in the front of the house and the technical services staff in the back of the house began to grapple with the change.

In his book *The End of Work* Jeremy Rifkin postulated that the new generation of powerful computers and the interconnections made possible by the Internet would lead to a shrinkage in the global workforce because information, the primary product of the post-industrial age, was now free from the constraints of paper and the need for people to move it back and forth. He also suggested that librarians along with middle managers, secretaries, bank tellers and wholesalers, among other middle-men, would be high-tech losers in the new information marketplace.

Technical services operations did indeed face the diminished workforce predicted by Rifkin, and they also faced the fact that much of the traditional work that they had done in the past still needed to be done. Books and issues of serials were still coming into libraries despite the inflationary hits most collections budgets had taken, so some new ideas were sorely needed.

In the November/December 1994 issue of the *OCLC Newsletter,* an article by Pam Kircher announced the new OCLC PromptCat service which was described as a new copy cataloging option. The new service was one product of OCLC's goal "to develop alternative methods for creating and delivering cataloging records, for increasing the availability of records for copy cataloging, and for providing more options for original cataloging." The service was based on first batch searching WorldCat (the OCLC On-line Union Catalog) for cataloging copy using book vendors' automated inventory records for non-serial materials. Subsequently, records for a library are output upon receipt of an automated inventory of materials shipped from the vendors to their client libraries. The article also announced that the new service had been tested in prototype at Michigan State University and The Ohio State University in 1993, and it would soon be available for the library clients of four book vendors: the Academic Book Center, Baker & Taylor, Blackwell North America and Yankee Book Peddler.

Some of Mr. Rifkin's "middle men" had come up with a very interesting idea.

We were ready for something new at the University of California, Berkeley. The Library at Berkeley had lost 30 percent of its professional and support staff between 1989 and 1994 as a result of three University-wide early retirement plans coupled with a blanket freeze on new hires. The Acquisition and Catalog Departments lost ten full-time employees in 1995 alone through attrition and reorganization within the Library for a savings of approximately $300,000 in the Library's operations budget. Further attrition in technical services staffing was inevitable because in a large group of 60 people, several resigned every year to take other jobs in the Bay Area or to relocate elsewhere. More attrition would definitely be a serious problem because there were absolutely no new funds to replace any Library staff.

In April 1995, Armanda Barone, supervisor of the Copy Cataloging Division, convened a task force consisting of cataloging, acquisitions, branch library and Library Systems Office staff to study the new Prompt-Cat service offered by OCLC. The task force examined the flow of the largest single group of materials, English language American trade publications, through the Acquisition and Catalog Departments and outlined how the new service might streamline the processing of these materials.

The task force recommended that we try the PromptCat service with two of our vendors, Academic Book Center and Yankee Book Peddler. We discovered that OCLC and the two vendors were as eager to try the new idea as we were. Since we were interested in a very early implementation of PromptCat, Ms. Barone and our systems staff worked extensively with the two vendors to insure that PromptCat catalog records, and our barcode and other local information in particular, arrived in the catalog in a consistent and uniform manner.

The workflow designed by the task force facilitates the electronic transfer of Berkeley's barcode numbers imbedded in the two vendors' inventory records to full cataloging records output from WorldCat. The cataloging records are then sent to Berkeley by FTP and loaded into GLADIS, our locally developed online catalog. A special circulation subroutine developed by our Library Systems Office automatically charges the records to Technical Services, and the public catalog display informs library patrons that the books are in the technical processing workflow. This is necessary because the bibliographic records always arrive several days to a week before the book shipments arrive from Yankee Book Peddler and Academic Book Center.

When the books arrive by UPS several days later, student employees initiate a discharge by wanding the barcode inserted in the book by the vendor which removes the processing charge. The circulation system also displays an abbreviated catalog record to the student processors allowing them to verify that the title on the book and in the record actually match. It also alerts them when incoming lower level records extracted from the WorldCat lack call numbers or lack subject headings outside the Library of Congress P class. These books are then forwarded to copy cataloging for evaluation and further attention.

After checking that the book and record match, the student employees apply spine labels derived from the Library of Congress call number in the record and send the books to be shelved in the main and branch libraries. All PromptCat processed materials are also property stamped and tattle-taped by the two vendors. The new workflow allows the general American trade books to be processed very efficiently by student employees and frees up support staff in receiving and copy cataloging to focus on more difficult foreign language materials. Approximately 14,000 monograph titles (13 percent) were processed through PromptCat in our initial year out of a total of 106,000 monograph titles cataloged.

In June 1995, the Acquisition and Catalog Departments were administratively merged into a single Technical Services Department. The merger facilitated the combination of the Processing Division, the acquisitions receiving unit, and the Copy Cataloging Division into a single division handling materials arriving through PromptCat as well other materials entering the cataloging process. The two departments remained on separate floors in the Doe Library building for a year while planning for a consolidated workplace progressed. In May 1996, the combined Technical Services Department moved to a single floor of the Moffitt Undergraduate Library. The facility is part of the new Doe/Moffitt complex which is connected by an underground stack area. We were fortunate to be able to consolidate our work space because it also enabled us to merge the serials cataloging and records maintenance units and to bring our original serial and monograph catalogers together in a single unit.

The task force which designed the PromptCat workflow realized early on that PromptCat would bring the same high percentage of incomplete Cataloging in Publication (CIP) records into the catalog as did the regular copy cataloging process. We planned from the outset to use a new parallel service from OCLC called OCLC Bibliographic Record Notification service to upgrade those CIP records. The service identifies each lower level record in WorldCat that had been delivered to Berkeley, and it automatically sends a higher level record when the CIP record is upgraded in OCLC. Several batches of upgraded records supplied by the service have been received in our Library Systems Office and await loading into the local catalog. The incoming higher level record will overlay the incomplete CIP record based on the OCLC record number in our local catalog without changing any location and call number information in holdings fields that had been assigned when the book was originally processed. Our planning task force thought that Bibliographic Record Notification was an essential adjunct to PromptCat because of the initially high percentage of CIP records. The problem has diminished greatly, however, since both the Academic Book Center and Yankee Book Peddler, among others, have launched efforts to upgrade CIP records.

The PromptCat and Bibliographic Record Notification services have allowed the Technical Services Department to maintain cataloging production at our traditional rate of over 100,000 titles per year using less expensive student employees in an era of greatly diminished staffing.

We have also recently begun a true shelf-ready beta test with OCLC in partnership with the Academic Book Center. After receiving an inventory list from Academic, OCLC outputs the matching OCLC-MARC records via PromptCat and immediately creates an electronic file of label records. The label records comprise the Library of Congress call numbers extracted from the OCLC-MARC records and the appropriate Berkeley locations. Academic receives the file via FTP at its facility in Portland, Oregon. Academic then produces spine labels and affixes them to the books about to be sent to Berkeley. The beta test has been in operation for only a short time, but we are very satisfied with the early results.

Another pilot service that we are exploring with OCLC is Repeat Search. The service features a periodic research of brief records representing a library's backlogged materials against WorldCat. When a matching record is identified, the library's holdings are set in the union catalog, and the library is notified via an electronic report. Backlog records which initially find no match in WorldCat are researched monthly, and any unmatched backlog records are returned to the library after a mutually agreed upon time period. While we have not added to our backlog in two years, Repeat Search will allow us to effectively deal with an older backlog of approximately 200,000 titles which had accumulated since the early 1980s.

Berkeley is, of course, not alone in suffering severe staff reductions and targeted reductions in technical services staff in particular. We have found it beneficial to develop strategic partnerships with OCLC and our library materials vendors to automate as much of the routine cataloging work as possible to make the most effective use of the remaining library staff. Services such as PromptCat, Bibliographic Record Notification and Repeat Search will move the bulk of the work of routine copy cataloging of American trade publications from library staff members and focus it instead on student employees and automated exchange of cataloging records.

It is clear from discussions with our vendors that libraries are asking them to expand their traditional business of selling books with cataloging and processing services, and they are quite willing to do this to remain competitive in the marketplace. We feel that the work thus far has been quite successful and certainly worth the development costs to the Berkeley library.

I feel that partnering with agencies outside the library to develop new services will become commonplace for library managers in the future. Technical services managers and catalogers already have the skills necessary to analyze and plan complicated bibliographic projects, such as retrospective conversion, based on MARC records. We learned at Berkeley that while we could not anticipate all the technical problems that might arise in implementing a service such as PromptCat, we had the skills to solve them together with our external partners, OCLC, Yankee Book Peddler, and the Academic Book Center.

Because of our diminished staff at Berkeley, a new staffing model for technical services is emerging. The professional catalogers are now working with more of the MARC bibliographic formats including manuscripts, visual materials and computer files. They are also tackling long-standing backlogs of unique archival materials as well as published materials from Third World countries and ephemeral publications in English and other European languages. Some of this work is grouped and organized on a time-limited project basis, and external funding is sought when appropriate. With more of the routine processing being handled by student employees and automated services, some of the remaining support staff are working in higher classifications doing original cataloging, archival processing and assisting the librarians in planning and implementing new services and procedures.

The technical services model that is emerging is one of a smaller, more flexible staff working to solve problems and develop systems across a broader range of technical services functions. That staff will be composed of a small core of professional librarians working with a group of more highly paid support staff managing systems and services that perform the routine work currently done in-house by lower paid support staff. Catalogers will be training paraprofessionals in original cataloging of print and electronic resources as well as archival processing; cataloging in several MARC formats; developing web-based manuals of procedures and policies; and learning completely new skills such as SGML and HTML coding and creating metadata for accessing electronic objects.

This model is also becoming evident in the collection development and public service departments at Berkeley as well: the much-reduced staff of collection development librarians is working with high level library assistants with subject and language expertise, and reference librarians are partnering with support staff to provide directional and catalog information services, as well as general bibliographic instruction including use of remote electronic resources and classes on navigating the Internet.

The most difficult challenge currently facing library managers is motivating supervisors and staff to become more flexible and to adapt to changes in the workplace. In positions at Harvard Law and Berkeley, I have observed staff apprehension toward procedural, organizational and environmental change. As a manager, I have organized several large planning efforts, the switch to AACR2 and the Library of Congress classification system at Harvard Law, and reengineering and relocating technical services at Berkeley. All these efforts involved broad staff involvement in a shared decision making process. I have found that while there was lively discussion and some creative thinking resulting in a generally agreed upon plan, staff often view the planning process as an end in itself completely distinct from any changes that might occur. This is the "It'll never happen" attitude brought about by a reluctance to change on the part of staff. This attitude often develops first among the staff who were the most involved in the planning process, possibly because they are in a better position to understand the scope of the changes that will come about. The attitude is also often reinforced by library administrators who are reluctant to sanction major changes in the workplace unless there is a consensus in favor of the change among the staff. In these situations, the manager is in the awkward position of having his planners saying "It'll never happen" while other staff are expecting a change and the library administration is expecting a consensus to develop. In these situations, all the manager's tact and resolve need to be called into play to initiate a change which is in the best interest of the library and to help the staff work out any problems that crop up along the way.

I have found that once the switch is flipped to initiate a change, it becomes old news in a matter of months. As staff see change happening in their positions and around them, more change becomes less threatening. They become accustomed to the manager's style in running the planning process, and they can see tangible benefits from the changes that have occurred. In my experience, there are always some staff members who are eager for a change in their working situation, but who choose to keep a low profile in the planning and change implementation process. It takes an insightful, attentive manager or supervisor to identify these people and bring them into the process after the controversy has died down.

At Berkeley, there was one very positive outcome of our well-publicized work with the PromptCat service: librarians from around the country began to call us to ask questions about our implementation and to visit Berkeley to see the actual workflow in place. The staff involved in the planning and implementation have spent time with the visitors discussing the problems they had encountered and the solutions that had been worked out with OCLC, Yankee Book Peddler and the Academic Book Center. After the visitors went home, the Berkeley staff were left with a sense of pride and accomplishment because of the recognition of their effort by others in the library profession.

In conclusion, the changes in the tasks of cataloging at Berkeley were necessary because the technical services staff was permanently shrunk by 30 percent through a series of University mandated early retirement programs. The technical services managers realized the need to reorganize the work and to seek new kinds of services from our traditional external partners, OCLC and our book vendors. The new relationships that we have forged with our old partners have allowed the Berkeley Library to continue to function in the current era of downsizing and cost containment in higher education. We feel that we are stronger for the effort, and we are in a better position to face further challenges in the future.

NOTE

Rifkin, Jeremy. 1995. *The End of Work*, New York: Putnam.

Reference Revolutions

Marilyn Gell Mason

Last year at a Summit of World Library Leaders held by the New York Public Library, 50 representatives of some of the largest libraries in the world met to discuss global library strategies for the 21st century. As one might expect, talk quickly turned to the challenges and opportunities provided by rapidly changing electronic technologies. In the course of the meeting one of the participants described the struggle of his library to help users gain better access to the now more than 36 million Web sites available worldwide (a number that is said to double every three months). He described the problem of getting hundreds, sometimes thousands, of "hits" when an individual tries to do even a simple search and talked about the need for libraries to apply knowledge classification schemes to electronic information. After he spoke, other members of the group reported dealing with the same problem and talked about their attempts to identify and classify databases that are especially helpful. Each of us, it seemed, was struggling with the same problem and each library was duplicating the efforts of every other. It was a familiar problem.

THE OCLC STORY

Thirty years ago, on July 5, 1967, ten leaders of academic institutions in the state of Ohio conspired to revolutionize libraries forever. These ten, three university presidents, three university vice presidents, and four university library directors met on the campus of Ohio State University to act

---

Marilyn Gell Mason is Director, Cleveland Public Library, Cleveland, OH.

[Haworth co-indexing entry note]: "Reference Revolutions." Mason, Marilyn Gell. Co-published simultaneously in *Journal of Library Administration* (The Haworth Press, Inc.) Vol. 25, No. 2/3, 1998, pp. 55-63; and: *OCLC 1967-1997: Thirty Years of Furthering Access to the World's Information* (ed: K. Wayne Smith) The Haworth Press, Inc., 1998, pp. 55-63. Single or multiple copies of this article are available for a fee from The Haworth Document Delivery Service [1-800-342-9678, 9:00 a.m. - 5:00 p.m. (EST). E-mail address: getinfo@haworthpressinc.com].

55

on a plan proposed by Frederick Gridley Kilgour, one of the library profession's great seminal thinkers. Kilgour had observed that libraries across the nation and around the world were spending millions of dollars doing the same work over and over again. At that time, the object of all the duplication was cataloging.

It is hard to remember now that until the last few decades every single library in the world was responsible for cataloging its own material. Even though the Library of Congress printed and sold catalog cards, each library, like every school at Harvard, was a tub on its own bottom. Every time a library received a new book it was responsible for verifying the author and title, assigning subject headings and a classification number, and printing and filing cards with the information in the library's card catalog (a monstrous and often error-ridden remnant of another time that has lately become the object of nostalgia in some quarters). At a cost of $30 to $60 per title, the price of all this duplication was enormous and libraries saw more and more of their resources going into cataloging, with less and less available to buy more titles or provide better reference services.

Kilgour believed that the solution to duplication was a shared effort that could be facilitated by information storage and retrieval systems that were becoming small enough and fast enough to handle the load. He believed that instead of waiting for the top-down efforts of the Library of Congress, which were often slow and cumbersome, libraries could function as a single unit held together by wires and electronic pulses. He believed that a title could be cataloged once, by a library in Texas or Massachusetts, and that the efforts of that library could then be shared with other libraries. Now we take the system that has become OCLC for granted, but in 1967 it was a revolutionary idea, and the articles of incorporation signed that fateful day in July were for a nonprofit organization called the Ohio College Library Center.

Four years later, on August 26, 1971, the Alden Library at Ohio University cataloged 133 books online and made history as the first library in the world to do online cataloging. Within a year Ohio University increased the number of titles cataloged by one third while reducing its cataloging staff by 17 positions. Kilgour's vision, that OCLC would increase access to information while reducing costs, was beginning to be realized.

As remarkable as that first year was, it was just the beginning, and while Ohio University was the first to use this remarkable new service, it was far from the last. By the end of 1980, when Kilgour stepped down as President of OCLC, the number of staff had grown from two to 500, the number of participating libraries had grown from the 54 academic libraries in Ohio to 2,300 libraries in all 50 states, and the bibliographic database went from zero to five million. Today the OCLC cataloging system handles over a billion transactions a year, with message traffic running as high as 110 messages a second. Today more than 24,000 libraries in 63 countries catalog more than 40 million books a year as well as other materials, such as maps, musical scores and sound recordings. The bibliographic database, now called WorldCat (the OCLC Online Union Catalog), contains nearly 38 million records and over 660 million location listings. It contains holdings in 377 languages and grows at the rate of two million original records per year. It is the single most consulted database in higher education.

As the database has grown, libraries have found other uses for it that go beyond cataloging. Foremost among them has been resource sharing. This year libraries will borrow over eight million items from each other using the information and support available through OCLC as an adjunct to WorldCat. This easy availability of often obscure material to anyone, anywhere, literally, on earth has revolutionized again the way we think about libraries.

THE REFERENCE STORY

Fred Kilgour's vision did not stop with cataloging. Shortly after it was clear that shared cataloging was a success, he began talking and writing about moving "beyond bibliography." He believed, and continues to believe, that OCLC can provide not just information about where to find information, but the information itself, the text of the book or article, the map, the recording, each delivered directly to the user. Initially, Kilgour's vision made librarians nervous. Some wondered aloud if OCLC would end up competing with libraries, competing with the very institutions it was established to serve. The debate did not last long as it soon became clear that in providing reference services OCLC was doing exactly what it had done so successfully in providing cataloging: it was enabling libraries to work together to do more than any one of them could do alone. Providing information that could be used directly by library users expanded conventional services in a way that strengthens libraries. Once again, OCLC was helping libraries use scarce resources cooperatively to provide access to more information for less money.

The OCLC FirstSearch service was introduced in 1991. It was designed to be used by both librarians and library patrons, a departure from the bibliographic databases. Like shared cataloging, FirstSearch started small, although small looked different it 1991 than it did in 1971. Initially six databases were mounted on FirstSearch: WorldCat; ERIC (Educational Resources Information Center); GPO Monthly Catalog; Consumers Index to Product Evaluations; BIOSIS/FS, a database created for FirstSearch that is derived from the Biological Abstracts portion of BIOSIS Previews; and MiniGeoRef, the most recent five years of GeoRef. Initially, FirstSearch was priced by the search, as were other, similar databases such as Dialog and Lexis/Nexis.

Today FirstSearch offers access to over 65 databases, including World-Cat, the New York Times and World Book Encyclopedia. It provides bibliographic information, abstracts or articles and full text. It is distributed through more than 10,000 libraries in 53 countries including China, Japan and Australia. The rate of use has climbed to 200,000 searches a day. In a recent issue of a quarterly report called *Information Market Indicators,* Martha Williams reports that FirstSearch is now the number one online provider of professional and scholarly databases. Additionally, in response to library requests, OCLC now provides subscription-based pricing for FirstSearch, enabling libraries to budget accurately and avoid becoming a victim to the success of the new service. (Many librarians feared that direct user access and success in getting needed information could result in almost unlimited charges with the continuation of a per-use pricing formula.) The availability of FirstSearch over the Internet has further reduced costs by removing incremental communications costs for many libraries in the United States while helping libraries outside the U.S. overcome international telecommunications barriers.

The most astonishing thing about FirstSearch is not its progress to date, but the certain knowledge that the reference revolution is still in its infancy. Like the early online catalog now known as WorldCat, growth is geometric, with FirstSearch now growing at the rate of 50 percent a year. If this trend continues, and there is no reason it should not, FirstSearch should itself account for over one billion searches a year in just seven more years. The reason this rate of growth is likely to continue is that, like WorldCat, FirstSearch provides a mechanism for libraries to do more cooperatively than any one library could do alone, and at a lower cost. In this case the duplication is not in the creation of catalog records, but in the negotiations with electronic producers of information. But there is much more to reference services than providing full text, and in these important developing areas libraries are finding themselves better able to do more by working cooperatively through OCLC than any one library could do on its own.

THE NEXT CHAPTER

The next stage of development for FirstSearch will see the introduction of OCLC FirstSearch Electronic Collections Online, Electronic Archiving, and Integrated Searching. In the recent summary of OCLC's strategic plan, called *Beyond 2000,* the problem is described succinctly:

"Despite rapid advances in electronic publishing and delivery technology, benefits to libraries and readers of scholarly journals have been slow in coming. Among the key reasons:

- High journal costs, and duplicate print and electronic costs, have been a barrier to progress.
- Archival Services, which are key to avoiding duplicate costs and realizing the economies of the electronic media, have not been forthcoming."

The new three-part initiative described in the strategic plan will be to:

- "Create a cost-effective, Web-based, scaleable delivery system for online journals and rapidly build a collection with a 'critical mass' of journals by topic areas.
- Create a suite of archival services encompassing long-term inexpensive storage, access for both content providers and third parties, scanning, indexing, and technology migration.
- Migrate toward integrated reference solutions embracing FirstSearch, SiteSearch and Electronic Collections Online to realize the vision of seamless access for the information user across a full range of information, including Web resources."

Electronic Collections Online will enable libraries to subscribe to both print and electronic journals from many publishers in a discipline and access them remotely through a single Web interface that will support searching through multiple journals and extensive browsing. Journals that libraries subscribe to will be loaded in their entirety either on or before publication date. In addition to current service, OCLC will provide continuing access to the archive of the journals to which they have subscribed. As more journals are issued in electronic form, this service will provide an easy and cost-effective way to manage large electronic collections.

Electronic Archiving will go beyond maintaining runs of journal holdings. As more and more materials are digitized, librarians are understandably concerned about document preservation and access into the future. The stability of electronic storage has not yet been demonstrated and to date changing technology has required continual shifts from one format to another. Many of us as individuals have experienced the loss of data stored on a disc that became so obsolete that no machine could read it any longer. Whole chunks of census data have been lost to the rapid migration of technology. To meet the challenge of preserving electronic documents or documents converted to an electronic format, OCLC is moving toward services that would support long-term, inexpensive storage for libraries individually and collectively. These services will include access for both content providers and users, scanning, indexing and technology migration. This cooperative approach to preservation and access is essential if libraries are to move beyond the current level of confidence in their ability to serve patrons in the future.

Integrated Searching will not only allow library users to search numerous FirstSearch databases simultaneously, but will also allow users to search both print and nonprint material. As any user of the World Wide Web knows, actually finding what you want from the welter of what is available can be a daunting task. Although books and other print documents are typically classified by subject, users of the Web are forced to rely on keyword searching, a process that mingles subjects that are unrelated and leaves the searcher with thousands of hits to sort through. Already OCLC has started work on a system (called the Scorpion Research Project) that will explore the possibility of automatically assigning hierarchical subject headings to many of the electronic items now available. This combination of automated retrieval and more conventional organizational structures has the potential for making electronic information more accessible and useable than it is today.

ELECTRONIC PUBLISHING–ANOTHER REVOLUTION?

Although not yet on the planning horizon, it is not hard to imagine that sometime in the next few years OCLC might enter the publishing arena in a big way. For years researchers have wondered out loud why commercial publishers should get rich by taking information from scholars for free while selling it back to university libraries for what some characterize as extortion prices. Independent electronic publishing has been touted as an alternative to commercial publishing but until recently has been inhibited both by the technical limitation in transmitting charts and other graphic material and the specter of an electronic free-for-all that could result if publication bypassed the peer review process. With the solution to the problem of capturing and transmitting graphics solved and made easily available on the Web, scientists and scholars are once again wondering what value commercial publishers bring to the distribution of scholarly information. Some are examining ways to keep the current review process without going through commercial publishers

Commercial publishers are beginning to offer their journals online. Elsevier, for instance, now makes all its 1,100 titles available electronically. In addition, smaller operations are beginning to make a mark. The Association of Research Libraries reports that the number of electronic journals has grown from fewer than 30 in 1991 to more than 300 in 1995. Still, the problem of pricing remains. The average cost of a scholarly journal has tripled since 1985, forcing research libraries to reduce subscriptions and shift resources away from other materials. Pricing of electronic journals by commercial publishers has not settled down but few expect to see any significant reduction in costs.

HighWire Press, a division of Stanford Libraries, has recently demonstrated what a university working alone can do. Starting in January 1995 with the publication of the *Journal of Biological Chemistry (JBC),* High-Wire is now nearly self-supporting, after only two years. More importantly, however, the HighWire effort has demonstrated that quality can be maintained in an electronic environment.

OCLC has also been successful in maintaining quality with its publication of *The Online Journal of Current Clinical Trials,* the world's first peer-reviewed online medical journal, which OCLC and the American Association for the Advancement of Science started in July 1992, and which is now published by Chapman & Hall.

It doesn't take much of a leap to imagine what might happen if OCLC, with its experience in networking, electronic distribution of information, electronic publishing, electronic archiving and integrated searching, joined forces with universities responsible for the creation of scholarly information. The result would be quicker, easier, cheaper access to scholarship around the world. It would be nothing less than a complete transformation of scholarly publishing. Researchers themselves would continue to write, edit and provide peer review for scholarly articles. The activity could be organized by scholars themselves through their universities, with universities having particularly strong departments in specific disciplines leading the way. OCLC could provide electronic publication and distribution using many of the systems already in place. Costs and benefits could be shared in much the same way that costs and benefits are shared through cooperative cataloging. The benefit to the scholar would be more immediate access to the latest research. The benefit to the university and the library would be a reduction in pricing.

Hard to imagine? It's probably no harder to imagine that academic institutions could collaborate to revolutionize the distribution of scholarly research than it was in 1967 for those ten academics in the state of Ohio to imagine that they could transform cataloging and thereby reduce costs. The goals are the same: speed up the flow of information and cut costs. The means are the same: use computer and communications technologies to link individuals and institutions. Even the motivation is the same: reduce wildly escalating costs that are overtaking the ability of libraries to provide a broad base of service. In 1967, it was cataloging costs that limited public service. In 30 years, OCLC has made it possible for libraries to reduce the cost to catalog one item from $30-$60 to less than two dollars. Today the cost of scholarly journals has ballooned out of control. In the last 30 years, catalog cards have become largely obsolete. Has the time now come for commercial, scholarly publishers to become obsolete?

Cooperation among research institutions through OCLC for the independent publication of scholarly material would do more than reduce costs. It would also speed up delivery, eliminate the need for interlibrary loan, eliminate many of the current copyright problems and enhance scholarship. Universities that were net contributors would be rewarded for their contributions, not penalized by the need to buy increasingly expensive journals.

THE OCLC MISSION

OCLC was founded in 1967 as a membership organization to serve libraries and library users for the following purposes:

- Maintain and operate a computerized library network
- Promote the evolution of libraries, library use, and librarianship
- Provide services for library users and libraries
- Increase availability of library resources to library patrons
- Reduce library costs
- Further ease of access to and use of the ever-expanding body of worldwide scientific, literary and educational knowledge and information

Throughout its 30-year history, OCLC has evolved to meet the needs of libraries using the latest technological capabilities. First it reduced cataloging costs and speeded up the delivery of quality cataloging. Building on that resource it used the existence of its enormous bibliographic database to encourage resource sharing. OCLC then moved beyond bibliography to provide not just information about information, but the information itself.

In the next few years it will add archiving and integrated searching, services that will further encourage the use of electronic information by providing confidence that documents can be found in the short run and preserved for posterity.

Cataloging was just the beginning, a tool to get the information we need. Reference has always been the goal. OCLC reference services are in their infancy. The one thing we can be sure of is that by working cooperatively, using the mechanism libraries have created through OCLC, libraries and their users can look forward to more information, faster, at a lower cost, now and tomorrow.

An Ongoing Revolution: Resource Sharing and OCLC

Kate Nevins

I still remember the first time I used the OCLC Interlibrary Loan Sub-system: the sun was shining, the birds were singing, and a simple OCLC system search revealed the correct bibliographic citation and holdings for a book requested by a patron. An online request form was sent easily to the holding libraries and the item appeared in my library within a week. All was truly right with the world. To understand my feelings of wonder, satisfaction and inner peace, you need to turn back in history to 1979, the year that OCLC automated and revolutionized interlibrary loan. Veteran interlibrary loan librarians can still remember the pre-OCLC days: complex searches for verification of elusive citations, laborious typing of ALA four-part forms to be mailed off to possible holding libraries, waiting weeks or even months for the item to arrive in the library to be placed in the patron's hands. Technological advances led to use of "round robin" circulation of needed items among libraries via teletype and TWX. Is it any wonder that I looked at OCLC Interlibrary Loan as the greatest thing since the Dewey Decimal Classification?

The introduction of the OCLC Interlibrary Loan System was revolutionary, and that OCLC revolution continues in resource sharing today.

THE 1979 REVOLUTION

It is almost quaint to look back at the time OCLC became widely used for interlibrary loan. The library literature from the late 1970s and early

Kate Nevins is Executive Director, Southeastern Library Network (SOLI-NET), Atlanta, GA.

[Haworth co-indexing entry note]: "An Ongoing Revolution: Resource Sharing and OCLC." Nevins, Kate. Co-published simultaneously in *Journal of Library Administration* (The Haworth Press, Inc.) Vol. 25, No. 2/3, 1998, pp. 65-71; and: *OCLC 1967-1997: Thirty Years of Furthering Access to the World's Information* (ed: K. Wayne Smith) The Haworth Press, Inc., 1998, pp. 65-71. Single or multiple copies of this article are available for a fee from The Haworth Document Delivery Service [1-800-342-9678, 9:00 a.m. - 5:00 p.m. (EST). E-mail address: getinfo@haworthpressinc.com].

1980s is full of analysis and discussion of the impact of OCLC's service on interlibrary loan operations. The topics and issues analyzed and debated may seem self-evident to us now, but at the time, use of non-automated interlibrary loan processes was pervasive, and a major change in thinking and practice was required. These changes took place in a number of areas: use of OCLC for verification and request transmittal, improved service to patrons, internal cost control, changes in work flow and changes in borrowing patterns.

OCLC for Verification and Request Transmittal

The basic interlibrary loan process includes three functions: verifying that the item exists, locating potential lenders and procuring the items. Printed tools such as the National Union Catalog and its Register of Additional Locations had long been the staples for item and potential lender verification, with various methods used to actually send the request to the potential lenders. These sources had several shortcomings for interlibrary loan purposes: main entry access only, small numbers of libraries submitting information and the time lag in publication, to name a few. Therefore, even before the availability of the OCLC Interlibrary Loan System, interlibrary loan librarians had begun using the bibliographic and holdings information created through the OCLC cataloging process for verification purposes. While still relying on paper-based methods to send the request to potential lenders, use of OCLC for verification introduced efficiencies and more effective service to patrons. In 1978, Ronald Rayman of Western Illinois University wrote, "Despite the fact that the (OCLC Interlibrary Loan) subsystem is not yet operational, it is apparent that OCLC is being widely used to facilitate interlibrary loans. The most obvious and practical application is the securing of locations." He goes on to note that OCLC verified requests have a successful fill rate of 81 percent.[1] With the introduction of the Interlibrary Loan System, many libraries began migrating to online interlibrary loan. The thought process of libraries considering this migration can be traced in articles such as "Special Report: OCLC Users Appraise the ILL Subsystem,"[2] "The Correct Use of Library Data Bases Can Improve Interlibrary Loan Efficiency,"[3] and "A Comparison of the OCLC Data Base and NUC for Bibliographic Checking."[4] Both within my library and on a consortia level, I took part in many meetings where we had detailed discussions of OCLC ILL system feasibility before we made the final decision to adopt it. I remember well the elation I felt when I realized I had punched my last tickertape for our TWX "Round Robin" borrowing wish list.

Improved Service to Patrons

The bottom line of interlibrary loan is the speed and accuracy with which patrons receive the information they need. Early articles describe the efficiency of the OCLC Interlibrary Loan Subsystem in these terms. A 1981 study by librarians at Queens College in New York showed a fill rate of 95 percent for OCLC-based requests, versus 76 percent and 84 percent for other methods. Turnaround time for OCLC-based requests was 16 days, versus 19 and 22 days for other methods.[5]

Internal Cost Control

Librarians were also interested in understanding the relative costs of non-automated and OCLC based interlibrary loan. A variety of studies were conducted, among them one by Bob Gorin at SUNY Stonybrook. He found that OCLC-based interlibrary loan cost $2.50 per item requested, vs. $5.59 per item requested over the TWX-based New York interlibrary loan network.[6] Other studies found similar results.[7]

Work Flow

Implementation of the OCLC Interlibrary Loan System required libraries to rethink the way they performed their functions and the necessary resources. This involved training in OCLC usage, availability of workstations, and changes in record keeping and management statistics.[8] I remember the delicate negotiations undertaken with my library's cataloging department to get scheduled time on the OCLC terminals in Technical Services for the Interlibrary Loan Department. Other libraries had these same struggles, as evidenced by this internal memo from the library at the Massachusetts Institute of Technology: "Last Friday the time of use of the OCLC terminal for interlibrary loan was cut from 30 to 15 minutes because the serials section needs more time. Fifteen minutes is really not enough time for interlibrary loan and we hope that, when the new terminal is installed, our time can be restored to 30 minutes, or possibly to 45 minutes."[9] And then there is this poignant advice, given by a librarian to his interlibrary loan colleagues: "If you don't have much terminal time, you'll get the most action if you transmit between 7:30 and 8:30 am."[10]

Borrowing Patterns

Traditionally, interlibrary loan protocols direct libraries to access resources located elsewhere in their geographic area, with state being the primary affiliation. If not available within a library's primary borrowing areas, material in other regions is accessed. The OCLC Interlibrary Loan System was designed to support this protocol by displaying holdings symbols sorted by state. Several interesting outcomes in borrowing patterns resulted from the adoption of the OCLC Interlibrary Loan System. First, state-based interlibrary loan programs were established or strengthened. State Libraries in many states, including Texas, Pennsylvania and Florida, built statewide programs using the OCLC Interlibrary Loan System. Second, while adhering to protocols for regional borrowing, libraries were able to successfully procure materials from a wide variety of lenders when necessary.[11] Third, while interlibrary loan still relied for its success on the rich collections of large libraries, the OCLC Interlibrary Loan System introduction saw the redistribution of many requests to smaller libraries whose collections had been largely outside of the lending mainstream.[12] I still remember the thrill I got when, working as ILL Librarian in a small college in upstate New York, we received and were able to fill a request from the interlibrary loan powerhouse, the University of Illinois. OCLC had made our collection accessible, and we were gratified to be able to provide, as well as request, materials from other libraries. Fourth, the OCLC Interlibrary Loan System led to a change in philosophy about borrowing partners. As Rayman wrote, "The commonality inherent in OCLC membership seems to foster, whether consciously or unconsciously, the conception that the OCLC database exists as a single, massive, commonly held library collection: borrowing from that collection through interlibrary loan seems a logical extension of that line of thought."[13]

At the time the OCLC Interlibrary Loan System was introduced, I was sure that we were at the very pinnacle of resource sharing systems. It had improved service to our patrons, helped control costs, led to new access patterns, and changed the very way we thought about interlibrary loan nationally. OCLC's interlibrary loan transaction volume has grown from 900,000 requests in its first year of operation to 8.1 million in fiscal 1996/97. This was a revolution, indeed. So, how could it possibly get any better?!

THE ONGOING REVOLUTION

In the nearly 20 years since OCLC introduced the Interlibrary Loan System, the changes it brought about have become institutionalized, and it takes an old timer like me to remember how revolutionary those advances were. Since then, both libraries and technology have changed dramatically, and these changes have resulted in new advances in the way we meet our patrons' information needs. OCLC has continued to be a major part of these advances. These advances include:

Internationalization

Just as internationalization has become so prevalent in daily life, so has librarianship experienced this trend. OCLC's membership now consists of libraries in 64 countries. A review of OCLC's newsletter illustrates the internationalization of resource sharing through such article titles as "PRISM ILL Goes Down Under,"[14] "OCLC Europe Reports Growing Interest in ILL,"[15] and "National Library of Canada Becomes OCLC ILL Supplier."[16]

Electronic Information Access

Libraries of all sizes and types are making increased use of both citation and full text electronic information. OCLC's resource sharing programs have expanded to include patron access to both types of electronic information. The OCLC FirstSearch service, introduced in 1991, is now accessed more than 35,000,000 times a year and use continues to grow. Ease of user access to citations is leading to higher demands for access to the cited materials.

Increased Efficiencies

In the face of increased demands and decreasing resources, libraries are working to increase the efficiencies of their operations. OCLC has brought this goal for libraries to the Interlibrary Loan System. There are several noteworthy enhancements that meet this goal. First, OCLC has developed the ILL Fee Management service which automatically tracks and reconciles ILL charges between libraries in order to reduce staff time allocated to process invoices and checks when libraries charge each other for interlibrary loan. Assuming an internal cost of $25 to libraries to generate or process an interlibrary loan related invoice, the ILL Fee Management service has saved libraries over 15 million dollars since its introduction in 1995.[17] Second, OCLC provides a computer-based training software package so that interlibrary loan staff can easily be trained in the System's operations. Particularly in academic libraries, where interlibrary loan departments rely on large numbers of part-time students, ease of training is important for efficient operations. Third, OCLC has developed a PC-based software package, the ILL Micro Enhancer, which frees staff from routine, repetitive interlibrary loan functions.

End User Borrowing

As a result of several factors–patron use of electronic information sources, the ubiquitous access to libraries' electronic Online Public Access Catalogs, the need for more efficient use of library staff time–there has been an increase in the initiation of interlibrary loan requests directly by patrons. OCLC has facilitated this important advance in several ways. First, patrons may initiate requests that are accurate and complete directly from electronic citations while using OCLC's FirstSearch service. These requests are then routed to the library's interlibrary loan staff for review before being forwarded to potential lenders. The Public Library of Cincinnati and Hamilton County reported that "The FirstSearch interlibrary loan feature . . . has decentralized interlibrary loan. . . . Patrons now have system-wide access to materials from across the country. Interlibrary loan is more convenient than ever before and has provided the means for better meeting patron demands for materials."[18] Second, OCLC has implemented the OCLC ILL Transfer program to support the transfer of patron-created ILL requests from libraries' local systems or campus E-mail systems to the OCLC Interlibrary Loan System. A librarian at Colorado State University has noted, "We handle between 25,000 and 28,000 requests per year, and that rate grows every month. . . . We couldn't begin to keep up with the volume without PRISM ILL (now OCLC ILL) Transfer."[19] Third, OCLC has established arrangements with a wide variety of document suppliers so that libraries and patrons may access these commercial providers as necessary. This both diverts the interlibrary loan burden, in part, from other libraries and provides a potential faster turnaround time for patrons. Documents supplied, which are accessible through OCLC, include *Engineering Information* and *The Genuine Article.*

These changes represent continued phases of the interlibrary loan revolution started with the introduction of the OCLC Interlibrary Loan System in 1979. Continued strides forward in internal library efficiencies and effectiveness of service to library patrons are the happy results of these OCLC capabilities.

CONCLUSION

Interlibrary Loan is a patron-centered activity in libraries. It is, therefore, appropriate to let a patron have the final word in this article. Author Doris Betts has spoken on the challenges of doing research for her books from a small town in North Carolina. In her view, she said, "The three greatest inventions of the Twentieth Century are the washing machine, the pill, and interlibrary loan."[20] High praise, indeed.

NOTES

1. Rayman, Ronald. 1978. "OCLC and Interlibrary Loan: A Preautomation Look." *RQ* Vol. 18 (Fall): 53.

2. "Special Report: OCLC Users Appraise the ILL Subsystem." 1980. *Library Journal* 105 (April 1): 767.

3. Thompson, Dorthea M. 1980. "The Correct Use of Library Databases Can Improve Interlibrary Loan Efficiency." *Journal of Academic Librarianship* 6 (May): 83.

4. "A Comparison of the OCLC Database and NUC for Bibliographic Checking." 1980. *Interlending Review* 8: 99.

5. Taler, Izabella. 1980. "Automated and Manual ILL: Time Effectiveness and Success Rate." *Information Technology in Libraries* 1 (September): 279.

6. "Special Report": 768.

7. Linsley, Laurie S. 1982. "Academic Libraries in an Interlibrary Loan Network." *College and Research Libraries* Vol. 43, Issue 4 (July): 292-9.

8. Nitecki, Danuta A. 1981. "Online Interlibrary Services: An Informal Comparison of Five Systems." *RQ* Vol. 20 (Spring): 7.

9. Sumner, Frances. 1976. "Use of OCLC Terminal for ILB Purposes." Internal Memo, Massachusetts Institute of Technology (September).

10. "Special Report": 769.

11. Nevins, Kate and Darryl Lang. 1993. "Interlibrary Loan–A Cooperative Effort Among OCLC Users." *Wilson Library Bulletin* Vol. 67 (February): 37.

12. DeGennaro, Richard. 1981. "Computer Network Systems: The Impact of Technology on Cooperative Interlending in the USA." *Interlending Review* 9:40.

13. Rayman: 53.

14. Burrows, Toby. 1995. "PRISM ILL Goes Down Under." *OCLC Newsletter* (November/December) No. 218: 18.

15. Barker, Liz. 1987. "OCLC Europe Reports Growing Interest in ILL." *OCLC Newsletter* (January) No. 166: 3.

16. OCLC. 1990. "National Library of Canada Becomes OCLC ILL Supplier for U.S. Libraries." *OCLC Newsletter* (November/December) No. 188: 8.

17. Mak, Collette. 1997. "IFM Cost Savings." Internal Memo, OCLC (May 22).

18. Fender, Kimber L. 1995. "Patron Initiated Interlibrary Loan Through First-Search: The Experience of the Public Library of Cincinnati and Hamilton County." *Journal of Interlibrary Loan, Document Delivery and Information Supply* 6: 45.

19. Wright, Becky. 1996. "ILL PRISM Transfer Continues to Streamline the Interlibrary Loan." *OCLC Newsletter* (March/April) No. 220: 30-31.

20. Betts, Doris. 1997. Author's Luncheon, SOLINET Annual Membership Meeting, Atlanta, GA (May 1).

Cooperation Among Research Libraries: The Committee on Institutional Cooperation

Thomas W. Shaughnessy

Although the history of cooperation among research libraries is characterized by numerous success stories, there are few, if any, collaborative ventures as successful as those of the Committee on Institutional Cooperation (CIC) libraries. The success of CIC library cooperation is remarkable from several perspectives. First, two private and 11 state-supported universities comprise the member libraries representing the University of Chicago, University of Illinois (2 campuses), Indiana University, University of Iowa, University of Michigan, Michigan State University, University of Minnesota, Northwestern University, The Ohio State University, Pennsylvania State University, Purdue University and the University of Wisconsin. Among the public universities, seven have land-grant missions. They are located in seven states, and the distance separating the members extends up to 1,200 miles. But, despite the diversity of the members and the distances, the commitment to a powerful vision of resource sharing and cooperation and the strong support of the chief academic officers who govern the consortium have enabled the CIC to succeed in ways that are truly remarkable.

The CIC was established in 1958. Its programs and activities include virtually all aspects of the academic enterprise except for intercollegiate athletics (the Big 10 organization fulfills this role). Throughout its 39-year history, nearly every academic unit on member campuses has enjoyed the

Thomas W. Shaughnessy is University Librarian, University of Minnesota, Minneapolis, MN.

[Haworth co-indexing entry note]: "Cooperation Among Research Libraries: The Committee on Institutional Cooperation." Shaughnessy, Thomas W. Co-published simultaneously in *Journal of Library Administration* (The Haworth Press, Inc.) Vol. 25, No. 2/3, 1998, pp. 73-85; and: *OCLC 1967-1997: Thirty Years of Furthering Access to the World's Information* (ed: K. Wayne Smith) The Haworth Press, Inc., 1998, pp. 73-85. Single or multiple copies of this article are available for a fee from The Haworth Document Delivery Service [1-800-342-9678, 9:00 a.m. - 5:00 p.m. (EST). E-mail address: getinfo@haworthpressinc.com].

benefits of the consortium. It is this spirit of cooperation among otherwise competitive universities that has produced the many successes of the CIC.

The programs of the CIC are guided by three basic principles: that no single institution can or should attempt to be all things to all people; that inter-institutional cooperation enables educational experimentation and progress on a scale beyond the capabilities of single institutions acting alone; and that voluntary cooperation fosters effective, concerted action while preserving both the autonomy and diversity of the participating institutions.[1]

These principles have taken root within the library component of the CIC, although in the decade following the creation of the CIC, discussions and the sharing of information among the library directors were the primary results. These discussions culminated in 1969 when a conference of CIC library directors and other staff was held to delineate a possible agenda for cooperation. Included in this agenda were the need for greater cooperative collection development and strategies for addressing the rising costs of scholarly materials.[2]

The 1970s saw the development of a special relationship between the CIC libraries and the Newberry Library, along with continued exploration of how to increase and extend interlibrary cooperation to move library programs and activities.

As the decade of the 1980s began, attention shifted to the need for preserving CIC library collections. Selected staff in a few of the member libraries set to work on advising the directors on possible strategies to address the problem. Two solutions were proposed: a coordinated program of microfilming and the deacidification of paper-based collections. In the mid-1980s a grant from the Sloan Foundation provided support for a conference on preservation. This meeting led to the formation of a task force on mass deacidification (1989). The task force produced a useful report, one that resonated not only within the consortium, but which also had an impact on other research libraries, archives and historical societies. While the use of mass deacidification of paper collections was not widely applied within the CIC for reasons of cost, several of the member libraries have proceeded to deacidify certain special collections by following the guidelines proposed by the task force.

During this period, other cooperative relationships were being developed and various projects tested. For example, meetings were held of librarians responsible for developing collections in the sciences and social sciences. There were regular reports on efforts to convert card catalogs to machine-readable form. There was a series of discussions on the need for online access to serials holdings information. Experiments were conducted on using telefacsimile software, developed by computing center staff at The Ohio State University, for document delivery. And a productive relationship was established between the CIC libraries and CICNET, an independent telecommunications network that provides Internet and other connectivity to the CIC universities.[3]

The libraries were also active during this period in seeking grants to support cooperative projects. Among the more notable successes in this area were a series of grants from the National Endowment for the Humanities for preservation microfilming. Activity in this important area continues to the present time.

The most significant advance in consortia cooperation, however, occurred in 1993 with the awarding of a $1.3 million grant from the U.S. Department of Education. This grant was made in response to a proposal to establish a Virtual Electronic Library (VEL) among the 13 member libraries. Although the VEL continues as a work-in-progress, it aims to provide seamless desktop access to the combined collections of the CIC libraries.

The Virtual Electronic Library project served to engage the member libraries in a far deeper and more focused manner. Several "list-servs" were developed to facilitate communication among library staffs concerning the project and regular meetings were scheduled among library automation directors, interlibrary loan librarians, collection development officers, and other staff. Various task forces were appointed to bring the project to fruition.

It soon became clear, however, that the VEL project had stimulated an entirely new approach to cooperation within the CIC with a concomitant need for strategic planning. In 1994, a draft plan was submitted to the library directors for approval. The plan included a vision for the library participants and a mission statement, and it delineated five broad goals, each of which was accompanied by specific objectives. The time frame proposed by the plan was five years, although provision was made for updating the plan annually. Once approved by the library directors, the plan was presented to the CIC chief academic officers for approval.

The chief academic officers were particularly impressed with the plan's vision and with the mission statement of the CIC libraries. The vision proposed in the plan is as follows:

> By the beginning of the 21st Century, the CIC libraries will have a cohesive consortial organization guided by a vision of the information resources in the CIC as a seamless whole, whether those resources are developed or owned individually or collectively. Through shared planning and action, the libraries and their patrons will have equal access to the total information resources of the CIC.

In addition, the libraries will provide the students, faculties, and staff of the CIC universities with access to comprehensive resources throughout the world. Through collective leadership and cooperative action each CIC library will realize extensive value-added services for its clienteles. The CIC libraries will be in the forefront of efforts to preserve, expand, and access both electronic information resources and traditional collections.[4]

The mission of the libraries is to attain the plan's vision by means of cooperation and collaboration that will advance the missions of the individual CIC libraries in their support of teaching, research, and service by:

- Creating–individually and collectively–new ways to fulfill the information needs of the faculties, students and staffs of the CIC universities
- Extending and enhancing the information resources and services available on each campus by providing equal access to complementary resources throughout the CIC
- Improving the collections, information resources, and services of the individual CIC libraries

The library directors, while strongly endorsing the vision and mission described in their strategic plan, also agreed that not every institution had to participate in every CIC program. This decision has enabled the consortium to make decisions more quickly–especially those relating to the joint licensing of electronic resources, as well as other areas.

The strategic plan and the consultative processes that led to its formulation, created a very ambitious action agenda for the libraries. This agenda was so broad in its ramifications and so demanding in terms of staff support, that the capabilities of the CIC central office were becoming strained. Clearly, a support staff within the CIC Executive Director's Office was needed.

CIC CENTER FOR LIBRARY INITIATIVES

In 1994, a proposal was submitted to the chief academic officers of the CIC universities to fund a center within the CIC which would be entirely devoted to realizing the goals of the CIC libraries. The proposal was accepted and each participating university agreed to contribute $10,000 per year for three years to support the center. It was in fall 1994 that the

Center for Library Initiatives (CLI) was established. Its function was defined as motivating, coordinating, communicating and facilitating the process of accomplishing the goals of the CIC libraries. The CLI was charged with providing staff support and coordinating the various functional teams and committees (collection development officers, library automation directors, heads of public services, etc.) that advance various aspects of the CIC libraries' agenda. The CLI Director, in addition to providing staff support to these groups, was further charged with providing leadership on issues of copyright and intellectual property, grants management, granting agency relations, and consortiumwide contracts with vendors.[5]

During its first two years, the CIC Center for Library Initiatives has played a vital role in achieving the ambitious vision of the CIC library directors, the creation of a single library resource, equally accessible to the students, faculty and staff of the CIC universities. The foundation for this vision is the technical infrastructure of the Virtual Electronic Library, which is currently under development. The collaboration that the CLI has fostered among the libraries has helped strengthen the organizational management of the consortium. Thanks to the VEL project, a much stronger sense of community, ownership, and responsibility for other cooperative projects has emerged.[6]

LEVERAGING INVESTMENTS IN LIBRARIES

Although the CIC libraries and their staff have long maintained a strong commitment to interlibrary collaboration and resource sharing, both the VEL project and the Center for Library Initiatives have made it possible to attain considerably higher and more effective levels of cooperation. The "compounding" effect of this accomplishment is quite extraordinary. To illustrate, the 13 member libraries contain more than 62 million volumes; they subscribe to some 550,000 serial titles; they employ some 3,000 staff; and they spend more than $280 million annually. Perhaps even more important is the CIC vision of making all of these resources available at the desktops of the students and faculty of the CIC universities.

One question that seems to regularly cross the minds of the CIC chief academic officers is whether it is possible to reduce investments in libraries because of such increased access to collections. In other words, why shouldn't the VEL project enable the member universities to reduce local investments in libraries? The answer is the fact that only by maintaining library budgets will the consortium remain strong. The VEL project will cause these investments to produce more access, to extend the use of library collections, and have a greater impact on university teaching and research. In effect, the collaborative programs of the CIC libraries are not designed to save money, but to enable the money put into libraries to have an impact far beyond the confines of a particular campus.

At the same time library investments are being leveraged by means of consortial licenses to various databases and electronic texts and by the sharing of staff expertise within the CIC. With regard to licensing, each library has a single point of contact for consortial licensing, a person known as the Electronic Resources Officer (ERO). All negotiations take place through the director of the CLI. Prior to any negotiations, the CLI director has a clear understanding of which libraries will participate in the licensing agreement and the parameters that define acceptable pricing. Finally, the mode of access to the electronic resource must be tested in advance and be acceptable to all parties before an agreement is signed. More than a dozen consortial licenses have been purchased by means of this approach. It is estimated that hundreds of thousands of dollars have been saved through consortial licenses.

The work of the EROs has been greatly facilitated by reports generated by another group of talented librarians, the Task Force on CIC Electronic Collection. Members of the task force represent various functions within their libraries and as a result, their recommendations are typically met with broad-based approval within the CIC libraries. It is this group, for example, that proposed the ERO structure, along with several other programmatic initiatives.

Investments in the CIC libraries have also been leveraged through the sharing of staff expertise. The presence of staff having national reputations in areas such as library automation and library systems at a few CIC libraries has worked to the benefit of all, particularly in terms of developing system specifications (for an interlibrary loan management system, for example), in achieving greater connectivity, and in interacting with the vendors of online systems.

In addition, staff who may not yet be recognized as national leaders often bring other skills and backgrounds to the task. Some, for example, have considerable technical skills; others bring programming experience; while still others are adept in interpreting the needs of library users. There is an enormous synergy flowing from these work groups and a well-developed culture for sharing ideas and insights, not all of which are CIC-related.

Similar advantages have accrued to the entire consortium thanks to the knowledge and ability of a few preservation officers and grant proposal writers. One of the more interesting experiments currently under way, however, is the sharing of a subject bibliographer between two CIC libraries. While employed on a full-time basis at one library, this person assists with collection development at another library. Four to five times each year, this librarian travels to the second library to meet with libraries and faculty in a particular discipline. Travel expenses are paid by the library visited, but no other funds are exchanged for this assistance. It remains to be seen whether this pilot project can be extended to other subject areas or to other specialized library operations.

Another example of the way in which the CIC libraries have capitalized on staff expertise is in the area of collaborative cataloging. Specifically, several of the libraries are helping to catalog the consortium's collection of electronic journals. These are currently stored in a server operated by CICNET, the consortium's Internet and networking provider. Similarly, several CIC libraries, in cooperation with the Center for Electronic Texts in the Humanities, are cataloging texts represented in the University of Chicago's ARTFL database.[7]

While the CIC libraries have made considerable progress in terms of retraining costs while increasing access to their retrospective collections and in particular to electronic resources via consortial licenses, they have been somewhat less successful in two critical areas. First, not all bibliographic records of titles owned by the CIC libraries are in machine-readable form. It is estimated that eight percent, almost five million titles within the consortium, remain to be converted. The result of this situation is that the collections included in this "non-reconned" group are not readily available for resource sharing. Progress is being made to address this situation, but it is slow, and as a result it will be some time before all of the consortium's bibliographic records will be available electronically.

In the second critical area, progress with respect to the prospective cooperative collection development has been slower than originally anticipated. In 1994, the CIC library directors acting on the recommendations of their chief collection development officers identified six subject areas for cooperative collection development. Most of the subjects selected focused on a single discipline, for example, physics, but others were less easily defined and in at least one instance was multi-disciplinary. As subject librarians became engaged in this process one of the serious problems that they had to confront was the lack of serials holdings data in convenient, readily accessible form. Nevertheless, good progress has been made in a number of areas, not the least of which has been the effective networking that is occurring on a regular basis among the bibliographers who have been involved in this effort. However, the participating libraries have not yet been able to claim victory in this critically important area.

MAXIMIZING THE USE OF INFORMATION RESOURCES

One of the key objectives for attaining the vision proposed for the CIC libraries is to expand the use of the 62 million volumes owned by the libraries, as well as the use of electronic resources. However, achieving this objective depends very heavily on the effectiveness of the VEL project.

Librarians within the CIC universities have initiated a number of projects which, when completed, will contribute to maximizing the use of the libraries' collections. Among these projects are:

- Determination of relative collection strengths by means of standardized shelf-lists counts
- Collaboration on the acquisition and licensing of electronic information resources, including electronic journals
- Collaboration on the joint storage (archiving) of electronic information
- Development of staff expertise in digital text conversion and encoding
- Collaboration on development of grant funding proposals for cooperative preservation of endangered materials
- Cooperation with publishers in the creation of a CIC electronic reference collection

All of these projects are under way and are indicative of the broad involvement of library staff in the work of the CIC.

IMPROVE DELIVERY OF INFORMATION
AND LIBRARY SERVICES

From a user perspective, perhaps the key indicator of the CIC libraries' success is the extent to which they have been able to achieve their strategic planning objective of improving the delivery of information and library services to CIC university students and faculty. While the VEL project certainly increases the likelihood for a wider range of accessible resources quickly and conveniently delivered, the VEL technology does not guarantee that this result will be forthcoming.

To set some specific targets that will, when accomplished, move the libraries towards this objective, the library directors agreed to:

- Jointly establish performance standards for lending and document delivery
- Explore various options for desk-top delivery of articles in electronic format to end users

- Establish a uniform loan period (4 weeks) for all CIC libraries
- Implement a joint contact with a delivery service for the transport of library materials ("returnables") among the CIC libraries
- Assume leadership for addressing copyright, licensing, and intellectual property issues

The CIC libraries' strategic plan proposed three additional objectives. The first addresses the need to develop the libraries' human resources. The second focuses on the need for economic and cost data. The third focuses on communication and the need to develop a more complete understanding both within the CIC and in national arenas of the nature and importance of interlibrary collaboration on the one hand, and its absolute necessity on the other.

THE VIRTUAL ELECTRONIC LIBRARY (VEL) PROJECT

The VEL project has become the foundation for most of the cooperative programs proposed by the CIC library directors. In fact, the VEL is the key ingredient for realizing the vision of the libraries–whose information resources will be seen as a seamless whole, regardless of their location or ownership.

A proposal for funding to establish a Virtual Electronic Library among the CIC universities was drafted in 1992 and submitted to the U.S. Department of Education. Subsequently, a grant of $1.2 million was awarded, payable over three years, with matching funds provided by the libraries.

One of the major technical challenges facing the libraries was how to link the four or five legacy online systems that the 13 member libraries were operating. Because the majority of the libraries were using NOTIS software, the CIC entered into negotiations with NOTIS to provide both Z39.50 and Z39.63 functionality and connect all of the libraries regardless of the systems that were in place. Shortly after NOTIS technical staff began work on finding a solution to the problem, NOTIS was purchased by Ameritech. After several months delay, Ameritech agreed to continue the partnership with the CIC and provide the necessary functionality. This task turned out to be far more challenging than Ameritech had anticipated, and after several months, the CIC elected to end the relationship. By this time, the CLI had been created, and it fell to the CLI's director to implement a new Request for Information (RFI) process. This process resulted in the selection of OCLC as a partner in an effort to build upon the OCLC WebZ software to achieve the desired outcome.[8]

The goals of the CIC's partnership with OCLC are to be achieved in two phases. Phase I includes a World Wide Web accessible interface into all CIC online catalogs and a patron request capability. Phase II includes a library management system for handling all interlibrary loan requests and functions, a transaction load-leveling capability and the generation of management information. The WebZ products, along with software to operate interlibrary loan servers which will be located in each library, will enable end users to request any item owned within the CIC libraries and allow for such access to take place without staff intervention. This latter feature will be a local option. Some libraries may elect to review all patron-initiated requests before they are sent, while others may not.

Apart from the interlibrary loan request functionality, the Virtual Electronic Library project includes a number of related objectives. These include an ability to:

- Integrate diverse local resources
- Maintain local control
- Provide a highly configurable environment
- Employ national and international standards
- Work across different online systems
- Provide desk top access for end-users
- Provide cost effective access to information
- Provide easy connectivity to libraries and networks that are outside of the CIC, as well as to commercial information providers
- Address copyright and other intellectual property concerns

The VEL Project has also served to bring about in most cases a closer relationship between libraries and campus computing centers. Just as the CIC library directors meet several times each year, so also do the CIC computing center directors or chief information officers. It is this latter group that provides the connectivity and infrastructure for the VEL. The CIOs have been particularly responsive to the library directors' concerns for greater database security and user authentication. The success of the VEL is of such importance to the CIOs that they have invited one of the CIC library automation directors to serve as a member of their strategic planning committee.

PREDICTORS OF SUCCESS

While it seems logical to assume that the various CIC library projects–joint licensing, Virtual Electronic Library, cooperative preservation projects, consortium-wide contract for document delivery, etc.–would be successful, what evidence exists that the students, faculty, and staff of the CIC universities are being better served? While user survey information does not yet exist (it would be somewhat premature to collect it since the VEL is still under development), there are several indications that most of these cooperative ventures have been successful and others hold considerable promise for success.

As of August 1996, for example, the CIC libraries realized a total cost savings of more than $700,000 by means of joint licensing of digital information products. By the end of the calendar year, it is estimated that these savings will exceed $1.2 million.

With respect to the preservation of library collections, the CIC libraries recently won a fourth grant ($1 million) from the National Endowment for the Humanities. While some NEH funding may have flowed to individual CIC libraries, there is no doubt that consortial proposals are far more successful than those of individual libraries.

Another, but perhaps indirect measure of success, is the fact that both the CIC university presidents and the chief academic officers have strongly supported the VEL project and have provided special funding for the CLI within the CIC office. These administrators appreciate the libraries' focus on existing strengths and their commitment to leverage investments in the libraries to provide richer collections and more service. While each participating library retains complete autonomy within the consortium, the federated model which has developed over the years facilitates joint action and new cooperative initiatives. In view of the diversity within the membership, this is probably the only model that would have any chance of success.

Finally, there are the results of sharing staff expertise. While difficult to measure with any precision, it is clear that sharing the abilities of highly specialized staff has had a major impact on the individual members' libraries and on the consortium's outcomes. Whether the topic is digital scanning, copyright, expertise with foreign languages or fields of study, integrated library systems, or vendor relations–to name but a few areas–the CIC libraries have benefited enormously from this pooling of specialized knowledge.

UNRESOLVED ISSUES AND CHALLENGES

By any measure, through cooperative efforts the CIC libraries have been able to improve services to their users, reduce costs and capitalize on their human resources. The full implementation of the Virtual Electronic Library project will bring about even greater campus access to CIC collections and information resources. There are, however, several factors that either can limit the consortium's success or strain collegial relationships.

First and foremost among the problem areas is intellectual property and fair use in the electronic environment. While this is an issue facing all libraries that wish to share electronic texts with other libraries, it is an issue that has the potential for severely limiting the CIC libraries' ability to achieve their vision.

A second issue is the ever present tension between institutional competitiveness and the commitment to cooperate and work together. The fact is that the CIC universities do compete for federal grants and research contracts, for outstanding faculty and for well-qualified graduate students. Sometimes the aspirations of an academic department may lead faculty in that department to insist on the development of local research collections versus relying on collections held by other libraries in the CIC. A corollary of this situation might be the insistence on having local subject specialists to both develop and interpret the collections. In such situations, the impetus toward resource sharing can be side-tracked by local academic politics.

The need for stronger database security systems and user authentication systems is another problem area. However, thanks to the support of the CIC's chief information officers, good progress is being made to address this matter.

Another question that needs to be more clearly addressed is the extent to which non-CIC libraries might participate in the consortium's programs and services. This is more of an issue for CIC Land Grant university libraries where there are well-established statewide expectations for access to their collections and services. A somewhat related question concerns the possible role of statewide or regional library networks in CIC library programs. Thus far, most of these questions have been addressed on an *ad hoc* basis, but eventually some policy guidelines may be needed.

The spirit of cooperation that has come to characterize the CIC libraries has given new meaning to resource sharing among research libraries. The pattern that they have established is being studied and copied by research libraries in North America as well as in several other countries. This article has attempted to provide an overview of some of the more salient components that have led to their success, along with some of the issues that continue to challenge these libraries as they set new standards for information access and inter-institutional collaboration.

NOTES

1. "The CIC Libraries: A History of Cooperation" (internal report). 1996. Urbana, IL. Committee on Institutional Cooperation.

2. *Ibid.*

3. *Ibid.*

4. "CIC Libraries' Strategic Plan" (internal report). 1996. Urbana, IL. Committee on Institutional Cooperation.

5. Allen, Barbara, and Roger G. Clark. August 16, 1996. "The CIC Center for Library Initiatives Self-Study and Evaluation" (unpublished). Urbana, IL. Committee on Institutional Cooperation.

6. *Ibid.*

7. *Ibid.*

8. "The CIC Virtual Electronic Library: Unifying Strategy for Collaborative Action" (CIC Homepage). 1997. Urbana, IL. Committee on Institutional Cooperation.

Context for Collaboration: Resource Sharing at the State Level

James A. Nelson

THE CONTEXT

Kentucky is an interesting and intriguing state for lots of reasons–the Presidents of both the Union and the Confederacy, Lincoln and Davis, came from this state, as did "The Great Compromiser," Alben Barkley. Legends of the Hatfields and McCoys tarnished the image of a proud people as did a mindless TV sitcom about life in the mountains where the world's first combined Library and Televillage service is being developed. To top it all off, the state's motto, "United We Stand, Divided We Fall" could decorate the flag of any library consortium or cooperative today.

There has been much going on in Kentucky over the last several years: much activity in trying to improve a struggling education system, a limited economic development effort, and the legacy of a bureaucracy which is underinvested in technology. The Kentucky Education Reform Act, KERA, was a landmark piece of legislation designed to completely over-haul the state's K-12 education system and while it didn't say much about libraries (except to allow for Library Instruction to be substituted for Moral Instruction–an interesting swap to be sure), it did drive kids to libraries in droves as they took on more self-directed learning and writing portfolios full of ideas garnered from books. It also committed the state to huge investments in technology. There may never be a final estimate, but

---

James A. Nelson is State Librarian and Commissioner, Kentucky Department for Libraries and Archives, Frankfort, KY.

[Haworth co-indexing entry note]: "Context for Collaboration: Resource Sharing at the State Level." Nelson, James A. Co-published simultaneously in *Journal of Library Administration* (The Haworth Press, Inc.) Vol. 25, No. 2/3, 1998, pp. 87-95; and: *OCLC 1967-1997: Thirty Years of Further-ing Access to the World's Information* (ed: K. Wayne Smith) The Haworth Press, Inc., 1998, pp. 87-95. Single or multiple copies of this article are available for a fee from The Haworth Document Delivery Service [1-800-342-9678, 9:00 a.m. - 5:00 p.m. (EST). E-mail address: getinfo@haworthpressinc.com].

87

numbers have run in the hundreds of millions of dollars (it has been estimated that the discounts driven by the 1996 Telecommunications Act and rulings of the Federal Communications Commission could save nearly $220 million).

In 1992, an ambitious effort to streamline Kentucky's economic development led to the formation of the Kentucky Economic Development Partnership: a statutorily-based initiative which would put this critical effort in the context of a strategic planning process with a board which would stabilize the leadership there. As that law was being deliberated and finalized, the Kentucky Library Network persuaded the Legislature to insert language in a section dealing with "statewide network for training and assistance" (KRS 154.10-100) which said "The network shall employ, to the greatest extent feasible, compatible hardware and software and common databases *and library and information services databases networks* [emphasis added] in order to insure a free flow of information and assistance among the components of the network." Discussions are currently under way between the Department for Libraries and Archives (administrator of KLN programs) and Kentucky Economic Development Cabinet to promote local use of network technologies for economic development, particularly through public libraries; and, a new initiative to put public access Internet workstations in every public library in the state.

In about the same time frame, the Kentucky General Assembly created The Long-Term Policy Research Center to help span the turnover of Kentucky's Governor every four years. This group set about developing a long-range Strategic Plan to guide program and budget development for the state. Goal 18 of that plan states that "Kentucky will develop a state-of-the-art technological infrastructure that complements its learning culture and bolsters its competitive position in the world economy." One of the "Indicators of Progress" for addressing that goal is "Percentage of libraries offering free access to on-line services." Then, in the second biennium of Governor Brereton Jones' term, a panel of public and private leaders from across the state was named to streamline state government and make it more responsive to the people. That panel, "The Governor's Commission on Quality and Efficiency," released a series of recommendations, and recommendation 75 stipulated that the Department for Libraries and Archives should be designated as the official point of access to state government information by public agencies and the general public.

In 1994, the state's technology commission was streamlined and strengthened to become The Kentucky Information Resource Management Commission; its mission is to guide the planning, deployment and management of information resources in Executive agencies and the public universities with links to local governments and the private sector. Two key developments coming out of this statewide collaborative system were the deployment of an interactive video classroom system called The Kentucky Telelinking Network (which should have about 200 classrooms by the end of 1998) and the Kentucky Information Highway. KIH is a statewide integrated backbone network composed of a consortium of local exchange carriers led by Bell South to provide very competitive rates for all state and local public agencies, including all schools, libraries and courthouses. The State Librarian serves on this commission by statute, a fact which gives the state's library community access to statewide technology development. In 1976-78, a period of much transition in state technology deployment, the State Librarian also served as Chair.

The pace quickened in Kentucky with the election of Governor Paul Patton, an engineer by education and training, and a former local official. He brought focus to the efforts to reengineer state government and more effectively utilize technology to do the state's business. In his first legislative session, Governor Patton was successful in obtaining over $100 million to fund his EMPOWER Kentucky initiative–the deepest and most ambitious business process reengineer effort in the country. The principle focus was on cost benefit activities with the goal of saving the state $50 million a year in real dollars. However, during the legislative deliberations on that program, the Public Library Section of the Kentucky Library Association got the language of the EMPOWER Kentucky bill amended to read, "The Secretary of the Executive Cabinet, the Redesign Steering Committee and the Secretary of the Finance and Administration Cabinet are urged to assign priority consideration to any proposal submitted for participation in the Technology Trust Fund by local public agencies through the Kentucky Department for Libraries and Archives for the purpose of providing technological access to world wide information sources to local communities and populations. For a proposal submitted by local libraries, the public services benefits shall be considered in lieu of showing demonstrable recurring cost savings."

This language, and the realization that there must be general public access to the information and services that EMPOWER Kentucky was making available through automating the operation of state government, led to the Public Library Internet initiative under the mandate of this high-level program. With state government on the way toward doing business differently, Governor Patton turned his attention to the state's Higher Education needs. A tough and widespread debate during a special session of the Legislature ended up with a new structure for Kentucky's post secondary education system–the four-year universities separated from the community colleges and technical schools. Part of the higher education debate focused on the concept of a "Virtual University" for Kentucky, utilizing the Kentucky Telelinking Network and the Kentucky Information Highway. As part of the deliberations on higher education, the public university library directors, affiliated as the State-Assisted Academic Libraries of Kentucky, made a parallel proposal for a "Virtual Library" and the Kentucky Library Association circulated a White Paper on the role libraries have in the Commonwealth.

The "Virtual Library" initiative is currently under way at this writing, but the key here is that the library community, in the context of the Kentucky Library Network, is expanding its use of the OCLC FirstSearch solution and working towards the eventual goal of using SiteSearch for access to all types of databases. As part of its move into their new 134,000-square-foot, state-of-the-art W.T. Young Library, the University of Kentucky has mounted SiteSearch as a resource for its students and faculty as well as the state's library community.

Another important contribution of EMPOWER Kentucky was the development of a "Commonwealth of Kentucky Strategic Information Technology Plan" which was done by a high level team of senior executive Information Resource Managers with the assistance of a consultant from the Deloitte & Touche Consulting Group. The State Librarian participated in this planning process as Chair of the KIRM Commission and its "Guiding Principles" are compatible with library development in the state:

1. Support the business objectives of the Commonwealth government
2. Conduct Commonwealth business electronically
3. Treat information as a strategic resource
4. View technology investments from an enterprise perspective
5. Ensure electronic access to information and services while maintaining privacy

This strategic plan will serve as a road map for a new Chief Information Officer position which will be the management structure for Kentucky State Government in coming years.

THE NETWORK

The foregoing prelude of "Context" is not just an effort to talk about the state of Kentucky. It is in large part the context for library development in this state which contributes to the uniqueness of The Kentucky Library Network, Kentucky's platform for information resource sharing, cooperative library services and OCLC services. KLN grew out of an initiative of the State Advisory Council on Libraries in 1980 (for more detail, see "KLN Inc.–Organizing for Resource Sharing in the 1990s").[1] Like many other library networks, KLN began as a microform and paper-based resource sharing organization, built a state database, and moved into the electronic age with a CD product which was, for many libraries, the only kind of automation they had experienced to date. It was the right thing for the times, and some libraries used it as an Online Public Access Catalog for checking their own collections.

Collaboration and a good mix of types of libraries is assured by the composition and organizational structure of the network. With more than 280 member institutions, the composition breaks out to be primarily public (45 percent), then evenly (about 18 percent each) for academic, school and special. The State Library, as the "corporate" library for state government, holds a special library membership, but it also serves as the operational and management arm of the network. Institutions join, pay dues and elect a Board, but staff at the Department for Libraries and Archives, in the State Library Services Division, carry out the programs. Funding, except for membership dues and income from meetings, also comes from the Department.

Even with a CD-based resource sharing system, KLN members used the world-wide OCLC for doing business. Several libraries were already members of OCLC, others joined, and the state brought the others in when the Group Access Capability was available. In this situation, much as is done in North Carolina, staff at the Department for Libraries and Archives serve as intermediaries between these "Selective Members" of the GAC and OCLC as well as SOLINET, thereby reducing workloads at the utility level and allowing pricing to stabilize at more reasonable levels. KLN contracts with SOLINET for much of its training, but a lot is done by teams of volunteers from the more sophisticated libraries who work with the others to achieve parity among network use.

Through a state and federally funded data conversion program, nearly one million records have been added to the state database, which stands, at this writing, at 3.2 million records and 8 million plus holdings. An interesting statistic here is that in this database are 1.8 million records which are owned by only one Kentucky institution. State protocols for borrowing and lending are established by KLN members working through the Board and "closest and smallest" has long been a priority to take some of the burden off the larger collections and to show how smaller libraries often have much to offer. The combinations of the data conversion program and these protocols have combined to make KLN a truly collaborative organization. There are 169 KLN members who have or are contributing records to the database, but every new member has to agree to actively participate in KLN activities so there is community membership by all. Of those contributing members, 68 are full OCLC cataloging members; 30 are Selective Members who contribute via a KDLA tapeloading service; and there are 71 who only contribute to the Kentucky Union List of Serials database.

The state Union Listing of serials at OCLC is managed by the University of Louisville through a contract by the Department for Libraries and Archives. At this writing, the Kentucky list includes 145,606 records and 151,408 holdings in the 169 contributing libraries. An earlier effort by the Department to get the smaller public libraries included in this listing service not only contributed records to the database, but it has assisted those libraries to keep their serial services up-to-date and helped address the "closest and smallest" protocol for this aspect of resource sharing. The SAALK libraries cooperated to sponsor an Ariel document transmission system (developed by the Research Library Group) to facilitate fax capacity, among their libraries, and the Department has been a contributing member of RLIN through its Kentucky Guide Project–to locate, describe and create access to archival holdings in the state.

In 1996, the Department launched a pilot project to test the value and desire for online database access and resource sharing for KLN members at the direction of its Union Database Committee. An extensive list of vendors was selected to receive the RFP for this pilot and the winning product was OCLC's FirstSearch. The pilot included 21 institutions, representing a cross section of KLN membership, and several options for how it would be used, including some "end user" testing. The Union Database Committee helped select the core set of databases to be used initially during the pilot period.

After KLN determined that FirstSearch was a good solution for an expanded resource sharing and information service program, all members were queried as to what their interests were in participating. The proposed funding for this phase of the service was built on a cost sharing concept with the Department for Libraries and Archives serving as the "anchor tenant" with a commitment of $80,000 towards the total cost of the database access. The other subscription fees were determined on the local "market"–the number of library patrons served by the library. Each library paid at least $300 and the amounts went up with the SAALK group contributing $65,000 together to underwrite a major portion of the total cost, which ran around $180,000, including training and Selective Member costs to KDLA. For this first true operating year of the program, which would run from October 1, 1996 through September 30, 1997, 121 KLN member institutions signed up. This group was composed of 22 academic, 77 public, 7 school, and 15 special libraries.

It was assumed that once this first year showed more about use patterns, a new formula could be developed based on actual use metrics, not service populations. The selection of databases for the core services was WorldCat (the OCLC Online Union Catalog), ArticleFirst, ContentsFirst, FastDoc, ERIC, GPO Monthly Catalog, MEDLINE, PapersFirst, ProceedingsFirst, NetFirst and EBSCO Masterfile. Each library had to sign an agreement which committed them to the term of the project, to paying telecommunications costs (except that KDLA continued costs related to ILL resource sharing of the Selective Users); agreement to pay the annual negotiated subscription fee for their library; and that they would receive free training, documentation and telephone support from KDLA, OCLC or SOLINET. Subset groups or consortia of KLN membership were allowed to negotiate their own subscription rates on databases not included in this core set and the SAALK group picked three more (Books in Print, the CINAHL nursing database and Modern Language Association's database) for their use, and not every institution uses every one of these. In short, there is enough flexibility in this approach to allow for sub-groups to add what they want and still keep the group discount capability for all KLN members.

After several months of use, the KLN Board was briefed by KDLA staff who monitored the use through OCLC statistics. The evidence was quite strong that the service population basis for estimating subscription fees almost mirrored the actual use, so the Board decided to keep the same type of fee structure in place for a second year, so that libraries could budget for this level of expenditure. One concern (and it is one all of these kinds of services face) is that while we know fees are always subject to change, one never knows exactly how much. It is in this critical area that OCLC and regional organizations like SOLINET can make critically important contributions to the library partnership–through negotiation and the bully pulpit they can do much to create affordable services in expanding markets. Nobody had devised real accurate costing mechanisms for a resource, information, which is unlike all others: it is not finite, in fact it expands; it can be used by many people at the same time; the costs are primarily up front and should drop with more users. In fact, the vendor community gets market penetration without having to market to the public. A good product is thus promoted by the libraries who serve the various publics.

THE FUTURE

With the context of what Kentucky is doing in education reform, economic development, business process reengineering through EMPOWER Kentucky, and its Public Library Internet Project, as well as a new Strategic Information Technology Plan, the work KLN has done in its migration from microform and paper to bits and bites positions the Kentucky library community well for a strong partnership role in the coming years. The collaborative and participatory organization which KLN has put in place provides a responsive infrastructure to support developments in all priority development work under way in this state. This is the only way services and information can be effectively delivered in an environment where the ubiquity of technology is obliterating geographic, political and programmatic boundaries. The old practice of "stovepipe applications" and top down command and control program management traditions simply will not stand up in this environment.

On the horizon, there is tremendous potential for an even stronger role for libraries in the context of developing state programs through Site-Search. This complex, sophisticated and extremely flexible solution to the universal need of a "common front end" needed for user-friendly access to information and services offers a huge opportunity for the library community to be a significant player in every program development priority in every state in the country. This is particularly critical in an era where Federal programs are shifting to state-administered strategies which can be more responsive to independent state needs. The evolution from the Library Services and Construction Act (an early leader in state-administered Federal programs) to the even more state-based Library Service and Technology Act underscores the importance of collaborative state level efforts like KLN.

At this writing, the possibility of an expanded use of SiteSearch is under discussion. Already envisioned as the keystone of an integrated and broadly accessible "Virtual Library" solution to the needs of the plans for a "Virtual University" as well as to meeting the needs of K-12 education reform efforts, now it is being considered as a "common front end" solution for access to state information and services as well. If this comes to be, it will be a shining example of how the library community can provide strong leadership for the rest of the country in effectively meeting the needs of an increasingly electronic environment. The strength of library organizations has always been the commitment to collaboration for the good of the greater whole. Also, libraries and library vendors have the professional expertise for designing and deploying information systems which make information more broadly accessible through user-friendly applications.

As Kentucky moves toward this new era of electronic access to and use of information and services, the work done by our library community will undergird future developments and will be a large reason for the success of our state in a global community. The products and services of OCLC, whose strength is in its membership and the technical research and development it has brought forth from this membership, will be central to state level solutions across the country. With this kind of expertise and capacity built at the national level, and the many varieties of state infrastructures in place around the country, we can look to a very promising future for all Americans; no matter where they might live.

NOTE

1. Nelson, James A. 1996. "KLN Inc.–Organizing for Resource Sharing in the 1990s." *The Bottom Line: Managing Library Finance* Vol. 9, No. 1: 24-7.

The University System
of Georgia's GALILEO

Merryll Penson

The University System of Georgia and OCLC are building an innovative electronic library called GALILEO, the GeorgiA LIbrary LEarning Online system. The new electronic library delivers bibliographic, abstract and full text information to more than 2,300 academic, public, technical and school libraries throughout the state. And it uses software and online services from OCLC to build local databases and to merge diverse databases into a seamless information resource accessible through a single World Wide Web based interface.

The result is a customized, virtual library for the students, teachers and faculty of Georgia's educational community, as well as increased efficiency in research, scholarship and academic achievement. Users access library holdings, journal databases, image collections, and reference resources using one interface, one search process and one desktop–whether in the library, laboratory, office or home. Their journey could take them to an electronic journal on the Web, to a database halfway around the world, or deep within their library's archives.

FACTORS THAT MADE GALILEO POSSIBLE

A collaborative project of the Board of Regents of the University System of Georgia, GALILEO went online in September 1995 with the

Merryll Penson is Associate University Librarian for Public Services, Ilah Dunlap Library, University of Georgia, Athens, GA.

[Haworth co-indexing entry note]: "The University System of Georgia's GALILEO." Penson, Merryll. Co-published simultaneously in *Journal of Library Administration* (The Haworth Press, Inc.) Vol. 25, No. 2/3, 1998, pp. 97-109; and: *OCLC 1967-1997: Thirty Years of Furthering Access to the World's Information* (ed: K. Wayne Smith) The Haworth Press, Inc., 1998, pp. 97-109. Single or multiple copies of this article are available for a fee from The Haworth Document Delivery Service [1-800-342-9678, 9:00 a.m. - 5:00 p.m. (EST). E-mail address: getinfo@haworthpressinc.com].

libraries of the 34 public colleges and universities of Georgia. It now includes an additional 36 private academic libraries; 370 public libraries that reach 157 counties and 56 regional headquarters; 33 technical school libraries; and some 1,855 school libraries. Fifty private K-12 schools will be invited to participate by July 1998.

Noting the creation and rapid growth of GALILEO, one Georgia legislator remarked "timing is everything." Three key factors came together at the right time to make GALILEO possible--cooperation, leadership and technology.

Cooperation

First, the cooperative framework needed to plan and implement a project as big as GALILEO was in place when the idea of a statewide electronic library was formally proposed. The Regents Academic Committee on Libraries (RACL), a University System committee made up of the library directors of the 34 system institutions, had been meeting for 30 years and had an impressive list of accomplishments. Examples of its cooperative efforts included: a joint borrower's card that lets users check out materials at another institution; an electronic union catalog housed at Georgia State University; support for automated library systems by DeKalb College and Georgia State University; and the sharing of databases mounted at Georgia State University and the University of Georgia that allows RACL members distributed access and reduced license fees. The long history of library cooperation made the concept of a shared, statewide electronic library achievable in many people's eyes.

Leadership

Second, Georgia had the right leadership in place at key levels of the higher education community to successfully support and fund the vision of a statewide electronic library.

Education was the top priority of Governor Zell Miller. In 1994, he established a state lottery to fund educational programs at all levels with special emphasis on new scholarships, technology development and pre-kindergarten programs. GALILEO's original funding came from lottery proceeds that supported technology development. The Governor's support of GALILEO meant statewide support for the project.

In the summer of 1994, Stephen Portch was named Chancellor of the University System of Georgia. One of his first decisions was to seek proposals for technology intensive and systemwide projects that would benefit all 34 institutions. This approach was a change for the University System of Georgia, where projects were typically funded institution by institution. Since the University System had funded few systemwide projects in the past, it was a bold step.

Dr. J.B. Mathews and Dr. Joan Ellifson, Vice Chancellor for Information Technology and Vice Chancellor for Academic Affairs for the University System of Georgia, respectively, also were very supportive of libraries. They played a significant role in Dr. Portch's selection of a library project as one of his special initiatives in educational technology development.

Finally, University System librarians were recognized as established leaders in information technology as a result of their involvement in state, regional, and national library organizations, including the Georgia Library Association, SOLINET (Southeastern Library Network), Southeastern Library Association, OCLC, and the American Library Association. They also were astute political leaders, having helped establish the annual Georgia Library Legislative Day where librarians and library trustees meet with the Georgia legislative members to discuss library issues and concerns across the state. In addition, they had networked with other information and education professionals to build support for libraries and technology. This collective leadership, from the Governor's desk to the reference desk, was essential to convincing key decision makers of the value of GALILEO and the impact it would have on their constituents.

Technology

The third key factor was technology. At long last, technology showed the promise of putting the power of information and education fully to work. The introduction of the World Wide Web, the newly released OCLC SiteSearch software, lower hardware and telecommunications costs, and increased availability of electronic databases and electronic full text all combined to make GALILEO doable. There remained some economic, cultural, legal and bureaucratic obstacles, but technology was no longer a barrier.

THE PROPOSAL

Defining the requirements of a statewide electronic library actually began in 1989, when Dr. Mathews established a subcommittee of the RACL library directors to advise him on library and technology matters.

This advisory committee established minimum standards for library automation systems, identified the need for retrospective conversion for more effective resource sharing and discussed possible electronic library scenarios. Consequently, when Dr. Portch issued a call for proposals in the summer of 1994 that would benefit all 34 public colleges and universities, there was already a consensus on the services and features that were most desirable for the University System libraries.

Under the auspices of the Vice Chancellor for Information and Instructional Technology, a proposal called "A Vision for One Statewide Library: GALILEO" was prepared in August 1994 that outlined six goals and that requested funding for eight central services and features.

The goals were:

- To ensure universal access to a core level of materials and information services for every student and faculty member in the University System of Georgia–regardless of geographic location, size of institution or mode of instructional delivery: traditional residential, off-campus, or distance learning
- To improve information services and support through increased resource sharing among University System libraries, thus providing a greater return on investment
- To provide the necessary information infrastructure so that all students in rural or metropolitan settings in the University System can be better prepared to function in an information society
- To enhance the quality of teaching, research and service by providing worldwide information resources to all faculty
- To ensure that adequate PeachNet bandwidth and statewide backbone are available to campuses to support library activities
- To place the University System in the forefront of library information technology, enhancing its reputation, along with PeachNet and distance education

The eight objectives, which supported the goals, were:

1. *Provide PeachNet access to all University System and off-campus center libraries.* Access to PeachNet was vital to all libraries in order to locate and retrieve information, share resources with other institutions, and support distance learning activities. Five system and approximately 25 off-campus center libraries did not yet have access to PeachNet.
2. *Provide the electronic full-text of core academic journals.* Most libraries never had been able to provide the approximately 1,500 core

academic journals that were required to support undergraduate instruction. Electronic access made the information equally accessible to system institutions and distance learning sites and avoided the duplicate costs of multiple acquisitions. Several vendors provide full text for half of these journals–they are continually adding more–and indexing and abstracts for all of them.

3. *Convert all University System card catalogs to computer format.* To facilitate locating and sharing library materials systemwide, card catalogs needed to be converted to computer format. Significant portions of each library's collection are unique within the University System. While most libraries in the System had begun converting their card catalogs to computer format, they had only partially completed the task.

4. *Provide automation for each system library.* An automated library system is essential to any academic library to support reference, circulation, acquisitions, and cataloging activities. Ten system libraries had not yet been able to afford an automated system.

5. *Support universal borrowing.* All University System students and faculty needed unimpeded access to materials held at any library. Universal borrowing required a central database of eligible borrowers, a courier service for books to be sent from one library to another, and a facsimile system for sharing copies of articles.

6. *Facilitate sharing of research journals.* Research journals are essential to university level institutions and to faculty conducting research throughout the University System. Students at all institutions deserved the opportunity to use these journals when involved in advanced projects. With a database loaded at the University of Georgia, students and faculty could review the contents of approximately 10,000 research journals, identify subscribers to the journals and initiate requests for copies of articles of interest.

7. *Provide electronic access to state census data.* The data contained in the U.S. Census pertaining to Georgia is of great potential use for research and instruction as well as for economic development, but the process of obtaining needed data was very cumbersome and obsolete. Funding was requested for hardware and software to provide online access via PeachNet to the most used portions of the U.S. census data.

8. *Distribute state publications electronically.* Under state law, the University of Georgia Libraries are responsible for acquiring and making available all publications of state agencies. Universal access supported instruction, research, and service activities at all Univer-

sity System institutions as well as providing a valuable public service. Funding was needed to acquire and maintain the hardware and software to scan, store and electronically distribute these publications.

The Chancellor embraced the goals and objects with considerable enthusiasm and made the proposal a major component in his request for new programs. The proposal was approved by the University System of Georgia and was sent to Governor Miller, who endorsed the concept and included it in his budget request for supplemental funds for fiscal year 1995 and for new funding in Fiscal year 1996.

PLANNING AND IMPLEMENTATION

As the proposal wended its way through the legislative process, the library directors and the Office of the Vice Chancellor for Instructional and Informational Technology began planning for the project in the event funding was approved.

In October 1994, RACL organized two groups: a Library Services Work Group and a Technical Services Work Group. The Library Services Work Group consisted of the existing RACL advisory subcommittee and made recommendations regarding library issues. The Technical Services Work Group, made up of systems staff, dealt with technical issues.

Subcommittees of one to 34 people worked on:

- Selection of databases
- Development of the GALILEO web page
- Automation issues
- Allocation of workstations
- PeachNet access
- Functionality of workstations
- Platform selection
- Networking
- Universal borrowing (courier service, centralized patron database, circulation, and ILL)
- Georgia publications and state census data
- Training
- Retrospective conversion.

A Steering Committee, made up of four presidents of University System institutions, along with several library directors and the Vice Chancellor for Information Technology, oversaw the entire planning effort. It discussed and reviewed recommendations from the various work groups, committees and subcommittees and provided progress reports to the Chancellor and University Presidents.

By the time the Georgia General Assembly approved the funding in March 1995, most of the planning was complete and many decisions had been made concerning hardware, software and databases.

Two server sites had been selected: one at the University of Georgia in Athens and one at Georgia State University in Atlanta. The University of Georgia site would use an IBM Power Parallel SP2, while Georgia State would use a Sun SparcServer 1000. These servers would host databases and provide a gateway to remote databases and resources.

OCLC's SiteSearch software was chosen as the search engine, primarily because it provided the same search engine as the OCLC FirstSearch service, an online reference service that offers more than 60 databases. Librarians in the University System had deemed access to FirstSearch a high priority, and SiteSearch provided a seamless link to FirstSearch. In addition, SiteSearch was fully compliant with the Z39.50 standard for open information systems. The software would allow libraries to build local databases, load commercially available databases locally, and to merge these seamlessly with remote databases under one World Wide Web interface for a single point of access. With SiteSearch, libraries can optimize the mix of local and remote databases and users literally won't be able to tell the difference. Furthermore, SiteSearch also provides tools which allow for the creation of web pages that are compatible with Netscape. These tools were used to develop the search screens and to allow ease of access to the Internet.

Two UMI databases were selected after considerable investigation and comparison. They were: Periodical Abstracts, Research II, a database that covers 1,600 journals in all fields and provides the full text of about 650, and ABI/INFORM, a database that covers about 1,000 journals in business and economics and provides the full text for about 500 journals. Together, these two databases provided indexing and abstracting for more than 2,600 titles and the full text for more than 1,100 of them.

Four hundred Pentium 75 machines, the latest and greatest at the time, were purchased and distributed to University System libraries, along with high quality laser printers.

To coincide with the beginning of fall quarter, RACL set a target date of late September 1995 as the implementation date for GALILEO. From March through August 1995, implementation began.

PeachNet, the statewide data communications network that links campuses to each other and to the Internet, was expanded to more than 80 routers and upgraded to T1 or T2 lines to handle the anticipated increase in traffic. Computer support staff networked campuses, adding libraries and additional computers. Prior to GALILEO, many campuses had limited or no web access and many library folks were operating in a DOS environment. Fax machines arrived late summer 1995.

SOLINET, the OCLC-affiliated regional network, provided training in Windows, Netscape, FirstSearch and the UMI databases. More than 50 sessions attended by about 1,000 participants were held at various sites across the state. A reference committee worked with SOLINET to produce common training materials for bibliographic instruction and library staff conducted numerous workshops for faculty and students throughout the system.

Retrospective conversion of approximately 585,000 records from 16 institutions began at OCLC, with SOLINET acting as project manager. Today, the main circulating collections for all University System libraries are in machine-readable form.

By late September, just 150 days after receiving funding, GALILEO was operational and 33 of the 34 institutions went online with public access to three databases: ABI/INFORM, Periodical Abstracts and Britannica Online. The 34th institution was delayed a month due to a construction project already scheduled in the library.

In November, a courier service began to improve ILL turnaround time and a major project to convert the University of Georgia's extensive map collection got under way. Efforts to convert government documents for Georgia's depository libraries also were initiated.

Private academic libraries were invited to participate. A Robert W. Woodruff Foundation grant helped provide funding for the private academic libraries already participating in the Atlanta area University Center consortium. Other private academic libraries organized themselves immediately to participate. The speed at which they organized for this purpose was unexpected, and this group has found other ways to cooperate as well.

In March 1996, the General Assembly provided funding to bring online 56 regional public library headquarters and 33 Technical Institutes across the state. A year later, the legislature provided funding for all county libraries (branches of the regional public libraries) and to all school districts. Training and technical support were provided to these groups as well.

GOVERNANCE

Ultimately, the Board of Regents has the responsibility for the GALILEO system. But with the system operational and with future development and expansion the primary concern, it was clear that a new governance structure was required. The presidents on the original steering committee no longer felt the need to participate, so RACL proposed a new structure that provided for some leadership continuity but also called for more participation by other members. Today, there is representation from all groups, including the private academic libraries, the technical school libraries, the public libraries, and the school libraries, as well as representatives from the two server sites. The new Steering Committee meets monthly to address policy issues and future directions. Anyone from any of the groups is welcome to attend the meetings, and minutes are distributed promptly.

The Office of Instructional and Information Technology of the Board of Regents provides the project director, who has responsibility for monitoring the budget, hiring staff, and working with contracts. The project director works with a Technical Committee to coordinate efforts between the two server sites, works out schedules for rollouts of new databases, and other technical matters. This committee meets monthly, often using the University System's GSAMS distance learning network.

RACL holds meetings twice a year and can revise GALILEO's governance as appropriate. For example, RACL proposed the use of an existing group which had been organized under the auspices of the Office of Public Library Services–GOLD (Georgia Online Database)–as the GALILEO User Group. GOLD now has representation on the Steering Committee. Flexibility has been the nature and strength of RACL; not much time is given to by-laws and parliamentary procedures. RACL values cooperation and the provision of information resources to users, and the focus remains there.

CURRENT STATUS

Databases

GALILEO has grown from providing access to three databases to more than 100 databases, along with over 2,000 journals in full text. Databases may be locally mounted on the servers at the University of Georgia or at Georgia State, or they may be accessed remotely through the OCLC First-Search service or through publisher web sites.

GALILEO makes the following databases available to all Georgia citizens:

- ABI/INFORM
- Census Data
- Dissertation Abstracts
- EBSCO Index Complete
- Business Dateline
- Collier's Encyclopedia
- ERIC
- Georgia Libraries Journal List
- Newspaper Abstracts.

In addition, all Georgia citizens have access to the Georgia Government Publications database, a database created using OCLC SiteSearch software. The software allows for the scanning and cataloging of full image documents. The database was created at the University of Georgia, the depository library for state publications, with the assistance of one GALILEO-funded library assistant.

A cooperative arrangement with GeorgiaNet, a state authority charged with marketing state information, provides free access to databases such as Attorney General's Office, the Georgia Code, State Agencies, Councils and Commissions, Administrative Rules and Regulations, records of the Georgia Secretary of State, and Legislative Services. Plans are for GALILEO to archive these resources.

Some databases have subsets to accommodate various levels of users. For example, while all have access to EBSCO Index Complete, access also is provided to EBSCO Middle School Search, EBSCO High School Search, EBSCO Primary/Elementary School Search, and EBSCO Health Search. Some databases, such as Academic Press Journals, Cambridge Scientific Abstracts, and Current Contents are accessible only to University System or private academic libraries. Some databases, such as the FirstSearch databases, are available only for academic and public libraries.

Menu screens are provided for each category of user group so they see a complete listing of databases. The screens also allow users to link to local resources that may not be a part of GALILEO. Passwords allow users to access databases remotely. For example, a student using his or her local library while home from school could enter a password to access Academic Press journals, yet the general users at the local library would not have that access.

In addition, GALILEO provides direct links to a Georgia Union Catalog and to Georgia library catalogs and web sites. It also provides links to various web sites that can directly support the educational process, such as THOMAS, the Federal Web Locator, and newspapers–including Georgia newspapers with web sites.

Staff and Support

GALILEO started with three staff members: two programmers and one library assistant to work on scanning the Georgia government publications. With an increasing number of users, the complexity of providing various menus, and the addition of numerous databases, more training, general support and technical assistance was required. The Office of Instructional and Informational Technology has recently instituted a GALILEO/PeachNet Service Center to provide assistance to GALILEO and PeachNet users. Additional programmers have been hired; however, much of the work of GALILEO is still contributed by University of Georgia, Georgia State University, the Office of Instructional and Informational Technology and other RACL members.

Assessment

Program assessment was a key element of the original proposal. Every University System library had established formal procedures to assess and evaluate its programs, usage, resources, and personnel in accordance with the Southern Association of Colleges and Schools criteria and University System assessment policies. GALILEO is being evaluated in the following ways:

Usage statistics. Programmers have designed the system to collect data on the number of hits, the number of searches by database and by institution, the number of full text retrievals; and the number of remote users. This allows everyone to know which databases are most used and by whom. It also indicates which libraries are the heavy users of GALILEO. At the September 1997 Board of Regents meeting, the Chancellor announced that GALILEO had reached its three millionth hit. Figure 1 presents a comparison of online statistics over three years.

FIGURE 1

	First full week of		
	Oct. 1995	Oct. 1996	Oct. 1997
Keyword searches	17,634	76,844	171,328
Fulltext displays	10,196	34,192	46,591
Citations displayed	34,124	134,818	300,412

Surveys. Feedback collected from a "Leave a Comment" button and an online user survey indicate that user satisfaction with GALILEO is high.
Legislative Review. At the Chancellor's request, librarians across the state invited local legislators to view GALILEO and to hear the benefits of GALILEO from faculty and students. Many legislators were pleased to see the benefits GALILEO provided to their constituents and that the project was accomplished in such a timely manner. Some were pleased to find they were cited in various databases!
Value. If libraries had to pay a per-search fee of 50 cents or per-article fee of $2.50 for the searches or full text articles retrieved by their users, many would spend more than their entire materials budget. Clearly this demonstrates the value of this collaborative model in making information available to all Georgia residents. As Governor Miller has stated, "GALILEO serves every one of our University System units with more resources than any of them could afford alone." In addition, libraries have found that their libraries are being used more due to GALILEO. Interlibrary loans, circulation and user traffic (door counts) have increased in many libraries.

FUTURE DIRECTIONS

To date, GALILEO enjoys strong political support, but as the economy, political priorities and players change, funding is less certain. Plans are under way to seek additional funding through grants or other collaborative efforts. Librarians must continue to inform funding decision makers that GALILEO was not designed to "save money" in order to reduce library budgets. Instead GALILEO has added value to existing resources by providing a wide range of information to all regardless of location or size, thus eliminating the information haves and have-nots. GALILEO has also fostered additional cooperative collection development efforts, particularly among the University System libraries. It has provided the impetus for the development of a single interconnected integrated library automation system for all University System libraries.

GALILEO continues to work with OCLC and is serving as a beta site for the new version of OCLC SiteSearch software written in JAVA programming language. This new version is expected to provide more powerful search capabilities for GALILEO users.

In addition to providing more databases and more full text resources, plans are under way to provide more Georgia information. More collaboration is expected with the GeorgiaNet authority in this arena. Consideration is being given to providing digital collections such as the 100 most important Georgia history titles published prior to 1920, or Georgia newspapers, or local history information available only to visits through special collections, or creating databases, such as Georgia Young Authors.

Student and faculty response to GALILEO has been tremendous. Immediately, user expectations increased. Once-reluctant faculty are now demanding more advanced workstations in their offices, so they can take advantage of GALILEO resources and get to the web. Students and faculty want more full text as well as more powerful machines. Reference librarians also have had to learn more about personal computers, as they seek ways to keep users from changing screens, loading their own software, wiping out hard drives, and printing every page they viewed.

Clearly, GALILEO has transformed libraries and is well on its way to becoming a statewide electronic library.

Telecommunications Options Connect OCLC and Libraries to the Future: The Co-Evolution of OCLC Connectivity Options and the Library Computing Environment

Marshall Breeding

INTRODUCTION

The success and sustained growth of OCLC reflects the value of OCLC's systems and services to libraries. OCLC's online products such as WorldCat (the OCLC Online Union Catalog) the Interlibrary Loan system, and the OCLC FirstSearch service have all proven themselves as valuable resources. The success of these resources to a large extent can be attributed to the effectiveness of the methods that OCLC provides for accessing its online systems. Its systems would be of little value if libraries lacked adequate access mechanisms.

I have heard OCLC staff say many times that the organization's central focus has always been on the content of its systems and services. Telecommunications has never been a goal in itself, but a necessary endeavor in

Marshall Breeding is Library Networks and Microcomputer Analyst, Vanderbilt University.

[Haworth co-indexing entry note]: "Telecommunications Options Connect OCLC and Libraries to the Future: The Co-Evolution of OCLC Connectivity Options and the Library Computing Environment." Breeding, Marshall. Co-published simultaneously in *Journal of Library Administration* (The Haworth Press, Inc.) Vol. 25, No. 2/3, 1998, pp. 111-128; and: *OCLC 1967-1997: Thirty Years of Furthering Access to the World's Information* (ed: K. Wayne Smith) The Haworth Press, Inc., 1998, pp. 111-128. Single or multiple copies of this article are available for a fee from The Haworth Document Delivery Service [1-800-342-9678, 9:00 a.m. - 5:00 p.m. (EST). E-mail address: getinfo@haworthpressinc.com].

which it must engage to support its primary interests. In this article, we explore the methods that OCLC has implemented over the course of time to make its services available to its member libraries. These access methods have evolved to keep pace with changes in the library computing environment.

At the time that OCLC began expanding its user base in the early 1970s, libraries lacked both the equipment to access such a system and the in-house technical expertise to install, configure and maintain complex telecommunications equipment. OCLC was extremely successful in creating access methods that could be managed under these conditions. Some of the characteristics of the network that OCLC constructed to meet the needs of this earlier library environment include:

- All equipment is provided by OCLC.
- Communications lines and all telecommunications equipment are installed by OCLC's designated agents.
- End-to-end support is provided from OCLC.
- Built-in diagnostics can isolate almost all error possibilities.
- Hardware is maintained by OCLC via its service agents.
- OCLC equipment does not interact with other systems except for record transfer.
- Proprietary networks and communications protocols.

Considerable time has elapsed since OCLC's beginnings. The computer and telecommunications industry has changed dramatically and the typical library computing environment has evolved accordingly. Today, the typical OCLC member library employs computers and networks and is involved with various types of automation projects and subscribes to a variety of electronic information resources. OCLC is but one of these resources and OCLC's role is to integrate their services into the library's computing environment. In contrast to the earlier model where OCLC assumed complete control and responsibility, a more modern approach might include these characteristics:

- Most computers that access OCLC are owned and maintained by the library.
- The library assumes more responsibility in providing support for its own communications environment, and OCLC services are but one feature of that environment.
- OCLC provides support only to the point at which it connects to the library's network.
- Failures within the library's network cannot be detected or corrected by OCLC.

- Library maintains its own computer and network hardware.
- OCLC's services are highly integrated with library's networks.
- OCLC follows industry-standard networking methods.

The latter approach ultimately offers a library more flexibility and control in the way it uses OCLC's services. Libraries that have adequate technical resources can take advantage of OCLC's newer access options as part of a more general goal of developing an enriched information environment. For libraries with more modest in-house computer expertise, OCLC will continue to offer its earlier more controlled environment for some time.

In order to provide highly reliable access to its services, OCLC developed and deployed an industrial-strength telecommunications network. From the time that OCLC began expanding its membership in the early 1970s, its network grew accordingly. This network used dedicated telecommunications circuits and proprietary communications protocols. In 1991, OCLC replaced this network with a totally new one based on X.25 packet switching technology, representing a $70 million investment. Today, OCLC is in the early stages of installing a new network based on frame relay telecommunications and TCP/IP protocols.

THE EVOLUTION OF OCLC'S ACCESS METHODS

When OCLC began deploying its services, libraries were largely not automated. For many libraries, OCLC terminals were their first computer equipment. Today, most libraries are steeped in automation. They operate library automation systems, provide access for their clients to the Internet, run CD-ROM networks, as well as many other computer-based systems. Less often does the library need OCLC to provide workstations and end-to-end connectivity, but rather to integrate its services into an existing library computing environment.

OCLC is constantly challenged to keep its telecommunications methods and options in step with the practices of the data communications industry and with the computer deployment trends in the typical library. As standards emerged, OCLC has reshaped its telecommunications network around those standards. While OCLC's original access methods were closed and proprietary, it has moved toward the use of standard network technologies.

OCLC's access methods must accommodate a wide range of library types. Whether the library be very large or very small, whether the library have one computer or hundreds, OCLC must offer a method for access compatible with its computing infrastructure, technical ability and fiscal means.

OCLC's telecommunications methods have evolved from a completely proprietary, self-contained network, where OCLC provided all equipment, to one that embraces local area network technologies and library-owned computer equipment. In the following section, I will examine how OCLC's access methods have evolved to accommodate changes in the library environment.

The Terminal-Based Environment

A look at OCLC's original environment puts the current environment into perspective. When WorldCat was started in 1971, it operated from a single Sigma 5 mainframe computer. OCLC's earliest network was based on static telecommunications links and data terminals. The original telecommunications network consisted of dedicated circuits between the host computers at OCLC in Columbus, Ohio, and each library. The earliest method for accessing WorldCat involved the use of daisy-chained terminals. The M100 block-mode terminal was introduced in 1973 and the M105 succeeded it in 1978. These terminals provided access to WorldCat, allowed the transfer of MARC records to local systems through an asynchronous serial port, and records could be printed on a serial printer. During this era, a common arrangement was for the library to pair an OCLC terminal with a terminal from its local system to transfer cataloging records. (An early OCLC terminal is on display in the Smithsonian Institution: Museum of American History, Information Age exhibit.)

These terminals communicated with OCLC's host computers through synchronous serial communications, using the proprietary "OCLC Library Linking Protocol." Synchronous communications involves an electronic clock pulse that controls the communications stream. The clock synchronizes the data communications process. The beginning and end of each data element is defined by its relation to the clock pulse. This contrasts with asynchronous communications, that uses no clock signal. With asynchronous communications, timing is not so critical. Stop bits and start bits define each data element, and the speed of the data transmission can be flexible. The synchronous communications used by OCLC relies on a polling process where each terminal in a group communicates with the host computer in turn.

The telecommunications links that connected libraries to OCLC's network were called multidrop lines. Originally 2400 bps, these links are now 9600 bps leased lines, provided by a long distance carrier. The multidrop line terminates in the library with a synchronous modem which in turn connects to a chain of synchronous devices, such as terminals. The early network used AT&T data circuits and Paradyne modems while OCLC's current network uses Sprint modems and data circuits. Each multidrop line can support up to 15 devices. Multiple multidrop lines are installed in libraries that require larger numbers of OCLC terminals. OCLC assesses a monthly network access charge for each multidrop line installed in a library.

Access Through Microcomputers

Data terminals such as the M100 and M105 are inherently single-purpose devices. These terminals were large and unruly devices, and it took two of them to perform basic cataloging operations–both an OCLC terminal and a local system terminal. The limitations of terminals eventually became more apparent. As more programmable devices emerged, the label "dumb terminal" was appropriately applied to these devices.

The microcomputer revolution began in 1981 with the introduction of the IBM PC. It was this system that first made microcomputer technology accessible to the business market. Earlier microcomputers were seen as experimental and mostly appropriate for hobbyists. But this microcomputer was developed and supported by the same company that had delivered large mainframe systems since the earliest days of computing. Many believed that microcomputers would bring radical changes to the business computing environment.

The IBM PC, however, lacked the ability to communicate directly on the OCLC network since its communications options included only asynchronous serial ports and parallel ports. Additional hardware and software would be needed to use PCs with the OCLC network.

In 1984, OCLC introduced the M300 workstation. This was basically an IBM PC equipped with a synchronous communications adapter. OCLC developed terminal emulation software for the M300 that allowed it to access WorldCat in much the same way as the M105 terminal. The keyboard layout of the PC differed in many ways from the M105 terminal, but the software remapped the keys. Bibliographic records could be transferred to a local system via the PC's built-in asynchronous serial port. Printing operated through standard parallel printers, which were much more popular than the serial printers required by the M105 terminals.

Over time PCs came into general use in libraries, and it became desirable for them to be able to use their own equipment. The purchase and support of OCLC-supplied equipment was a financial burden for many libraries. But the requirement for the synchronous communications adapter severely hampered the ability to integrate PCs into the OCLC network. The synchronous adapter was sensitive to timing issues and required hardware interrupts and an input/output address. These factors led OCLC to allow only M300 Workstations on its network and not allow library-supplied computers to be equipped with these adapters and connected to the network.

The M300 was but the first microcomputer-based access station offered by OCLC. This original device was based on the 8-bit Intel 8088 microprocessor. As this microcomputer family evolved, OCLC's workstations have kept pace. OCLC has offered workstations based on each of the Intel processors: the 8088, the 80286, the 80386, the 486, and the Pentium.

OCLC Communications Controller: Native Access for PC-Based Workstations

In 1988, OCLC introduced the Communications Controller, which allowed up to eight devices to access OCLC through asynchronous serial communications. This meant that PCs could access OCLC through their native serial ports without the use of an asynchronous adapter. For the first time, libraries could use a generic PC as a dedicated computer on OCLC's network without any special hardware. OCLC assesses the same monthly communications charge for each active port of a Communications Controller as it does for a dedicated terminal.

The communications controller itself was a PC with an asynchronous communications adapter and a multi-port asynchronous adapter. It ran software that controlled the flow of data from each of the devices attached to the asynchronous ports to the synchronous network. Through its own synchronous adapter, the Communications Controller connects to a multidrop line. Figure 1 illustrates a Communications Controller on a multidrop line.

The Communications Controller provided access for a variety of asynchronous devices. In addition to OCLC's own microcomputer workstations, libraries could connect their own microcomputers, saving the additional expense and maintenance costs associated with OCLC-supplied equipment. Increasingly, libraries are used to providing their own support for microcomputers and want the flexibility of doing so for OCLC access stations. The Communications Controller also supported asynchronous ASCII terminals. These devices had somewhat limited functionality, but were very economical.

Network Access to OCLC Through the Communications Controller

While the Communications Controller was designed to provide dedicated access to microcomputer workstations, there are a number of ways

The Cataloger's Workstation and OCLC Services

One of the models for providing a computer environment for technical processing is the "cataloger's workstation." Such a computer environment would include access to all the systems, services, and information tools required to perform technical services tasks. Some of the systems included on a cataloger's workstation would be access to the library's local online system, access to OCLC and other bibliographic resources, access to Internet-based services, and information resources such as the Cataloger's Desktop software from Library of Congress. The general principle of the cataloger's workstation is that all these resources be available to each person's individual computer rather than having staff go to other computers to get access. For OCLC Cataloging, the traditional access method involved was having a set of dedicated computers that technical services staff all share. This arrangement usually meant that staff had to take turns doing OCLC work and had to use this resource according to a set schedule. In a cataloger's workstation environment, access to OCLC would be available at any time, though it would be expected that each person would use these resources judiciously. The cataloger's workstation involves providing part-time access to a large number of computers rather than providing full-time access to a smaller number of shared stations.

The key to the implementation of the cataloger's workstation involves providing access to all the various resources through a local area network. Three different methods can be used to provide access to OCLC services through a LAN. These include network gateways to the OCLC Communications Controller, the OCLC's Telecommunications Linking Program, and the Dedicated TCP/IP Access to OCLC.

to provide a more cost-effective distributed access to OCLC using this device. The traditional configuration involves a cable that connects the serial port of the PC with one of the asynchronous ports of the Communications Controller. There is a one-to-one relationship between the number of computers that can access OCLC and the number of active ports on the Communications Controller. While this configuration is well suited for creating dedicated access stations that can be shared by a number of users,

FIGURE 1

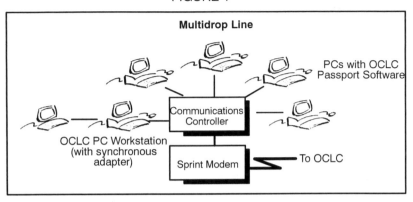

it is not conducive for providing part-time access to OCLC to a larger number of computers, following the Cataloger's Workstation model, for example. While it would be possible to string serial cables to each PC to provide part-time access and pay for an active Communications Controller port, this would not be a financially efficient model. Given the monthly charges associated with each active port on a Communications Controller, libraries must do all they can to maximize their use. The economic factor of maximizing use of OCLC ports, the desire to provide access to the largest number of computers possible, as well as the deployment of local area networks within libraries, led to the development of methods to integrate Communications Controllers into the network environment.

One of the earliest methods that emerged to distribute the use of Communications Controller ports involved terminal servers. With this model, each active port of the Communications Controller was connected to a port on a terminal server. The terminal server was then configured to offer the data on the port as a service to other devices on the network. Likewise each computer in the library that was to provide access to OCLC had a cable that attached its serial port to a terminal server. When one of these computers needed to access OCLC, it would issue the commands to request the service, and a virtual connection would be established between this PC and one of the Communications Controller ports, if there was one available. This arrangement allowed a much greater number of computers in the library to have potential access to OCLC than there were active Communications Controller ports. The number of simultaneous sessions was limited by the number of active Communications Controller ports. Depending on the workflow patterns of the library, each port could support from 2-4 actual users. Libraries might still choose to dedicate some ports to full-time use to accommodate special needs such as interlibrary loan offices, and other situations that use OCLC continuously.

The use of terminal servers to distribute access to the Communications Controller predated OCLC official support to network access methods. Libraries implemented these arrangements at their own risk, knowing that OCLC's support goes only as far as the Communications Controller. Any failures of the terminal servers, microcomputers, or any other part of the environment were the responsibility of the library.

Vanderbilt University implemented this type of OCLC access beginning about 1988. Not only were we at Vanderbilt able to gain distributed access to OCLC through the terminal server arrangement, we were also able to combine access to OCLC and our NOTIS system through a single microcomputer. Today, it is expected that computer users will access multiple systems though multitasking environments such as Windows. But in the DOS environment, this was not a trivial accomplishment. We connected the ports of an IBM 7171 asynchronous protocol converter to the same type of terminal servers so that library stations could also access NOTIS. We also attached each of the two serial ports of the PC to terminal servers, so that one could connect to OCLC and the other to NOTIS. A communications package (Mirror from Softclone, Inc.) provided both the terminal emulation and the task-switching environment. This software allowed itself and one other program to operate in the computer's memory at the same time. The user would press the designated hot key to toggle between the two programs. A NOTIS session would operate in the main communications program, and the OCLC terminal software was loaded as the secondary application. The user could instantly toggle between OCLC and NOTIS on the screen with a single key press. We also added a third serial port to the PC so that records could be exported to NOTIS through their Generic Transfer and Overlay (GTO) gateway. While this was a very cumbersome arrangement in many ways, it proved at the time to be a very effective means to creating a multi-purpose technical services workstation. This would not have been an affordable venture without the component that allowed us to share and distribute the use of each OCLC Communications Controller port.[1]

OCLC also developed methods by which libraries could integrate OCLC Communications Controllers into their networks. While terminal servers offer some capabilities for accessing online systems, local area networks (LANs) are far more efficient and powerful resource sharing environments. In a LAN, each microcomputer is equipped with a network interface card (NIC), usually either an Ethernet or Token Ring card. Through this one network connection, a large variety of services can be provided to the computer. Disk storage on a file server, access to shared printers, electronic mail, and access to various online systems are typically available on a LAN. In a library environment, one of the desirable options on a LAN would involve access to OCLC.

The Communications Controller can be integrated into a LAN to provide OCLC services to networked library computers. There are a number of different types of communications servers and gateways that can be connected to the asynchronous port of the OCLC Communications Controller to provide network access to OCLC. The main problem, however, lies in getting the terminal software to expect the OCLC session to operate from the computer's network card rather than from the asynchronous serial port. This problem was solved in 1992 when OCLC released Version 2 of Passport software which included support for a set of network drivers. The LAN drivers provided with Passport included those for Novell Asynchronous Server Interface/Novell Asynchronous Communication Server (NASI/NACS), NetBIOS, TCP/IP, and one for a generic one for BIOS Interrupt 14.

Providing LAN access to the Communications Controller through this approach involves creating an asynchronous gateway on the network and latching up its ports to those on the OCLC Communications Controller. For those with NetWare networks, Novell offered a product called the Novell Asynchronous Communication Server (NACS). This software ran in a computer that had a network card and a multi-serial port adapter. Each NACS port connects to an OCLC Communications Controller port. To access OCLC in this environment, Passport is configured with the Novell Asynchronous Interface (NASI) LAN driver. This environment allows a much larger number of library computers to have part-time access to OCLC. The number of active Communication Controller/NACS ports limits the number of computers that can access OCLC simultaneously. Details on the implementation of this model of access can be seen in Breeding (1992).[2] For those with TCP/IP networks, a terminal server can be used in place of the NACS. For access in this environment, Passport would be configured to use the TCP/IP LAN driver. Figure 2 illustrates how the Communications Controller can be integrated into a TCP/IP network through a terminal server. LAN access to OCLC was originally developed for the DOS version of Passport and this capability continues to be part of Passport for Windows.

At Vanderbilt University, we implemented networked access to OCLC through a set of NACS after a LAN was implemented in the library to replace the earlier terminal server environment.

FIGURE 2

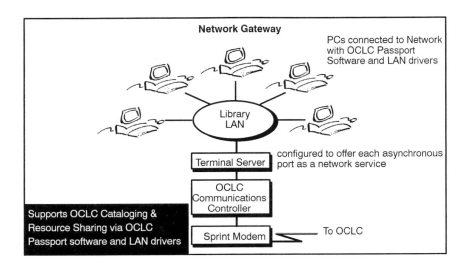

INTERNET ACCESS

Since 1995, OCLC has offered access to its cataloging and resource sharing services via the Internet. This access method was established after a successful 9-month trial. For many libraries, this approach allows them to take advantage of their existing Internet connection to replace or supplement other access methods. To access the OCLC system via the Internet, library computers must connect to a local area network that supports TCP/IP protocols and use Passport for Windows with its built-in TCP/IP drivers. The computer must also have installed a TCP/IP network stack that is Winsock-compliant. This is the same network software required to support the Netscape Navigator, Microsoft Internet Explorer and other web browsers, so most computers are likely to be properly equipped. The library's network must connect to the Internet, either directly, or via a campus or corporate network.

Connecting to the OCLC system via the Internet does not eliminate communication charges. OCLC assesses a per-minute connection fee for Cataloging and Resource Sharing over the Internet. For libraries with extensive OCLC access needs, it may be cost-effective to use other connectivity methods.

The main drawback of Internet access to OCLC services involves performance and reliability. OCLC built its private network to be extremely reliable and to offer consistent performance levels. The infrastructure of its network is well-balanced with the number of actual users. OCLC maintains over a 99.8 percent reliability rate on its network. Such is not always the case with the Internet. Service interruptions and periods of performance degradation are unfortunately much too common on the Internet. Many libraries prefer to maintain dedicated links to OCLC's private network for their production cataloging environment to avoid the vagaries of Internet access. Libraries with dedicated OCLC access can use Internet access to supplement the OCLC access during busy periods, and can use Internet access in the event of a service interruption on the dedicated network.

TLP

In 1992, OCLC introduced a totally new approach to providing access to its services called the Telecommunications Linking Project, or simply TLP. The previous access methods involved the use of OCLC-supplied equipment of various sorts, while TLP relies almost completely on library-supplied equipment. Through TLP, the library connects its existing TCP/IP network to OCLC's X.25 network via a 56 Kbps telecommunications link and a router that translates between these two network protocols. OCLC need not provide any hardware or other communications equipment to the library. The library provides the router which provides access to the TLP link.

A TLP implementation provides a fixed number of virtual circuits between the library's network and OCLC's systems. The number of virtual circuits represents the number of sessions that can be open simultaneously with OCLC services. All computers on the library's network are eligible for OCLC access, provided they have the right network software and access to Passport. TLP accommodates a very dispersed model of OCLC access, which contrasts with the other methods that concentrate OCLC use to dedicated terminal or microcomputer stations. Through TLP, as well as the other methods described above that provide access to OCLC on a network, it is possible to provide access to OCLC services to all library computers.

On the library side, TLP relies on a standard networking environment, usually TCP/IP. The library will have a local area network and all computers that access OCLC services must connect to the network. For TCP/IP networks, users' computers must have TCP/IP network software. While it is possible to use the DOS Passport to access OCLC services in a TLP network, Passport for Windows is the ideal method. Passport for Windows is a standard Winsock-compliant application, and will operate on any computer that has been equipped with TCP/IP network software. A number of products are available that provide the required TCP/IP environment for Windows 3.x, and some are available at little or no cost. Windows95 and Windows NT Workstations come with this capability built in.

The workstation environment required to use TLP is developing in most libraries. The overwhelming trend in networking is toward a TCP/IP-based network. Access to the Internet and the development of "Intranets" requires integrating TCP/IP software into an organization's desktop computers. Since Passport for Windows uses exactly the same network environment for desktop computers as programs such as Netscape's Navigator and Microsoft's Internet Explorer, TLP is quite consistent with the network developments that are going on in libraries anyway.

One of the limitations of TLP is its primary orientation toward Windows-based computers. In many ways this is not a major limitation since this is the dominant computer platform. DOS-based computers can be configured to access TLP, though in most cases it is much easier to implement Windows. OCLC offers software (LAN drivers) that will allow DOS Passport to operate with TCP/IP networks, but it is somewhat complicated to install. OCLC offered Passport only for DOS and Windows computers, and is ending support of the DOS version on January 1, 1998. At about the same time that TLP was made available, OCLC also released a product called Gateway. This software runs on a Unix computer and provides access to OCLC to computers that cannot run Passport. Through Gateway, libraries could allow their Macintosh computers and Unix-based workstations to access OCLC.

The router used for TLP will have at least two interfaces, a serial interface with connects to the Sprint modem via a V.35 serial cable. The router's Ethernet interface connects to the library's network. The router is then configured to perform a translation between the X.25 protocol and TCP/IP. Cisco's routers that operate the Enterprise version of its Internetwork Operating System (IOS) have this capability. When configuring the router, an IP address is assigned to the router's Ethernet interface, and a second address is used for the X.25 translation. It is this latter address that one uses to connect to OCLC. Figure 3 illustrates the TLP connection method.

One of the disadvantages of TLP involves its cost. The 56 Kbps X.25 telecommunications link required for a TLP implementation costs about as much as 4-5 9600 bps multidrop lines. TLP targets the larger libraries that would otherwise need four or more multidrop lines to support their OCLC access needs.

FIGURE 3

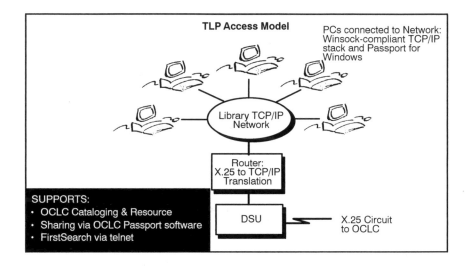

TLP Access Model

PCs connected to Network: Winsock-compliant TCP/IP stack and Passport for Windows

Library TCP/IP Network

Router: X.25 to TCP/IP Translation

SUPPORTS:
- OCLC Cataloging & Resource
- Sharing via OCLC Passport software
- FirstSearch via telnet

DSU

X.25 Circuit to OCLC

DEDICATED TCP/IP

OCLC's most recent development in telecommunications methods involves a product called Dedicated TCP/IP. This access method resembles TLP, but uses more up-to-date data communications methods. This new service relies on frame relay packet-switching technology and native TCP/IP network protocols rather than the proprietary OCLC Protocol over the X.25 packet-switched network.

OCLC Dedicated TCP/IP service is not Internet access, it is a virtual private network and can only be used to connect with OCLC services. Libraries that have Internet access may want to consider OCLC's Dedicated TCP/IP service to avoid the hourly connect fees that OCLC charges for access to its services via the Internet. Libraries can fairly easily calculate the break-even point between the number of hours of Internet access to OCLC versus the cost of maintaining a Dedicated TCP/IP line. Depending on the quality of the library's existing Internet connection, it is likely that OCLC Dedicated TCP/IP service will be more reliable and offer more consistent response time. The Internet is subject to unpredictable failures and degradation in performance during peak periods is common.

From the library's perspective, Dedicated TCP/IP works much like TLP. The library must have a LAN with support for TCP/IP network protocols for each PC that will access OCLC. The library must provide a router port or intelligent switch port (routing functionality must be available and supported). OCLC will install its own router that will interface with the library's router. Passport for Windows will be the primary access software for OCLC Cataloging and Resource Sharing, while telnet, Web browsers, and Z39.50 clients can be used to access other OCLC services such as FirstSearch. Figure 4 illustrates the Dedicated TCP/IP access method.

Dedicated TCP/IP offers several advantages over TLP. Frame Relay is a more efficient telecommunications protocol than X.25. For the relatively low-speed lines used by OCLC, frame relay is the optimum technology. While ATM (Asynchronous Transmission Mode) is generally considered the best switching technology for high-speed networking, the frame relay operates most efficiently for applications in the modest 56 Kbps to 256 Kbps range. While the initial deployment of OCLC's Dedicated TCP/IP service will operate via frame relay services, migration to ATM would be relatively easy should bandwidth needs increase dramatically. Such migration would be transparent to the end user.

Dedicated TCP/IP should be more cost-effective than TLP. I noted above a library must replace at least 4 to 5 multidrop lines with a single TLP line to break even in cost. OCLC has recently announced pricing for this service and the pricing for three or more workstation libraries is the

FIGURE 4

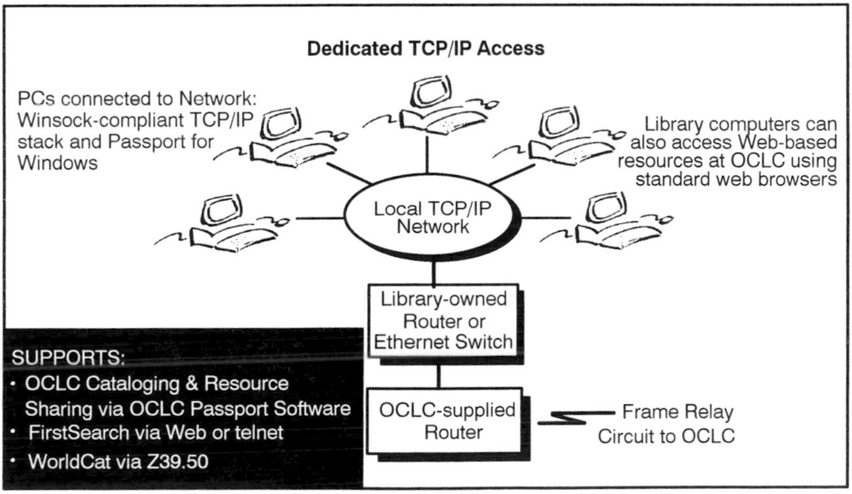

Dedicated TCP/IP Access

PCs connected to Network: Winsock-compliant TCP/IP stack and Passport for Windows

Library computers can also access Web-based resources at OCLC using standard web browsers

Local TCP/IP Network

Library-owned Router or Ethernet Switch

SUPPORTS:
· OCLC Cataloging & Resource Sharing via OCLC Passport Software
· FirstSearch via Web or telnet
· WorldCat via Z39.50

OCLC-supplied Router

Frame Relay Circuit to OCLC

same as they would pay for multidrop. This cost difference makes network access to OCLC accessible to smaller libraries.

A wider array of OCLC services can be supported through Dedicated TCP/IP. One of the recent developments in OCLC services involves Z39.50 access to WorldCat. This service relies inherently on TCP/IP and cannot easily work over TLP connections, but will be supported in the Dedicated TCP/IP service. Libraries may access any of OCLC's Web-based services through this method, including FirstSearch, OCLC First-Search Electronic Collections Online, and other OCLC Web servers including the OCLC Home Page. As OCLC migrates more of its services to a Web-based environment and as libraries deploy networks that support TCP/IP protocols, the Dedicated TCP/IP service will be the ideal access method.

OCLC's Dedicated TCP/IP service fits well into the current evolution of technologies. Even though the field test of the Dedicated TCP/IP service has just begun, this access method promises to greatly simplify the process of gaining access to OCLC's services for both large and small libraries.

DIAL TCP/IP ACCESS

Since 1974, OCLC has offered some sort of dial-up access to its system for computers and terminals equipped with a modem, through a standard telephone line (see Table 1). Many OCLC member libraries cannot afford to have dedicated terminals and prefer to access OCLC services through the dial-up method and pay an hourly connect charge. The OCLC Terminal Software, the DOS version of Passport, and Passport for Windows each were designed to support dial-up access in addition to equipment directly connected to the OCLC network. Computers can use other terminal emulation software to connect to OCLC services, but only OCLC's software can fully support features such as diacritics. OCLC offers dial-up access through value-added networks such as Compuserve as well as through its own dial-in servers. This dial-up service operates over an asynchronous serial terminal emulation session.

In conjunction with the Dedicated TCP/IP service, OCLC also plans a dial-up version of TCP/IP access. It has become common for computers to use SLIP or PPP software to connect to Internet Service Providers, corporate networks or campus networks. This software does not rely on a serial terminal session with a host computer, but rather establishes a TCP/IP network link with a remote network. This link operates much the same way as a LAN connection, but uses a modem and a telephone line rather

TABLE 1

Chronology of OCLC's telecommunications developments

1971	OCLC Online System began on a single Sigma 5 computer
1972	Use of the Spiras LTE Terminals
1973	Introduction of the M100 Terminal
1974	Dial Access
1978	Introduction of the M105 Terminal
1984	M300 Workstation
1989	First Tandem computer: Database Processor
1979	OCLC Online System expanded to four Sigma 9 computers
1979	A second Tandem computer added as Network Supervisor
1980	All computer equipment moved from facility near Ohio State to new headquarters on Frantz Road
1988	Introduction of Communications Controller–up to 8 asynchronous connections
1989	First OCLC System reached its largest configuration, with 17 Sigmas and 64 Tandem computers
1990	New OCLC system implemented on Tandem computers
1991	(Nov 26) OCLC completes the installation of its new X.25 packet-switched telecommunications network, a $70 million project
1992	Transfer of cataloging operation to new OCLC system complete
1992	(December) Cut-over of the ILL system to new OCLC system complete
1992	TLP (Telecommunications Linking Project) available
1992	Passport for DOS 2.0 with LAN drivers: NACS/NASI, NetBIOS, TCP/IP and BIOS Interrupt 14
1994	(October) Internet access to OCLC trial
1994	(December 17) The last of the Sigma computers was decommissioned
1995	(February 1) Internet Access to OCLC available to all OCLC customers
1997	14 percent of OCLC cataloging and resource sharing operates through the Internet access
1997	(August) OCLC offers Dial TCP/IP Access
1997	(year end) OCLC will offer Dedicated TCP/IP Access

than a network interface connected to a high-speed computer network. With current modem technologies, computers can communicate on a SLIP/PPP session at speeds up to 56 Kbps. OCLC's dial-up TCP/IP service will offer access to the same information products as the Dedicated TCP/IP service. This new service is completely consistent with the general trend in computer use toward PPP-based dial-up methods.

SUMMARY

OCLC's access options have generally kept pace with the evolving trends in the telecommunications industry and the library computing environment. In the absence of any existing technical infrastructure in libraries, OCLC initially delivered a complete access solution. As libraries deployed microcomputers and developed networks, OCLC has offered access methods consistent with such an environment. The overwhelming trend in the current era involves the Internet and Intranets. It seems that the whole computing world is rapidly converging on TCP/IP networks and Web-based information systems. OCLC has worked quickly to re-orient its networking paradigm towards these technologies. Libraries will do well to embrace these new access methods to make OCLC services just another component in their network-based information environment. Proprietary access methods and equipment are remnants of the past, while integrated networks rich in information resources are required for libraries to be the information leaders of the future.

NOTES

1. Breeding, Marshall. 1991. "Multipurpose technical services workstations: Access to NOTIS/OCLC/GTO with a single microcomputer." *Library Hi-Tech*, Issue 35, Vol. 9, No. 3: 69-81.

2. Breeding, Marshall. 1992. "OCLC Connectivity: Current Models, Network Integration, and Future Directions" *OCLC Micro* 8:4 (August): 28-36.

OCLC in Asia Pacific

Min-min Chang

INTRODUCTION

In his classic work on automation, John Diebold noted that any important technological innovation brings about three phases of change. In the first we simply do better what we did yesterday . . . The second phase begins when, as a result of technological innovation, we find the tasks themselves changing . . . The third phase is a change in society itself as a result of this transformation.

K. Wayne Smith, President and Chief Executive Officer of OCLC, wrote the above in 1993. Smith thought at that time that "in libraries, we are still largely in that first phase . . . but we are rapidly moving into the second."[1]

Reviewing the changes that technology has brought into libraries in the past four years, it is obvious that we are well into the second phase. There are indications that even the third phase–change in the library itself–has begun.

Established as the Ohio College Library Center in 1967, OCLC has grown into the largest computer and telecommunication network of libraries and information centers in the world: more than 24,000 libraries in 63 counties and territories are OCLC users in 1997. In the past three decades, OCLC has provided a series of computer-based products and services to libraries and has played a key role in facilitating cooperation and resource sharing among libraries on a global scale. The OCLC Online

---

Min-min Chang is University Librarian, Hong Kong University of Science and Technology.

[Haworth co-indexing entry note]: "OCLC in Asia Pacific." Chang, Min-min. Co-published simultaneously in *Journal of Library Administration* (The Haworth Press, Inc.) Vol. 25, No. 2/3, 1998, pp. 129-140; and: *OCLC 1967-1997: Thirty Years of Furthering Access to the World's Information* (ed: K. Wayne Smith) The Haworth Press, Inc., 1998, pp. 129-140. Single or multiple copies of this article are available for a fee from The Haworth Document Delivery Service [1-800-342-9678, 9:00 a.m. - 5:00 p.m. (EST). E-mail address: getinfo@haworthpressinc.com].

Union Catalog and Shared Cataloging System began revolutionizing technical services operations in American libraries 25 years ago; today, the FirstSearch service is revolutionizing public services in libraries worldwide. OCLC has altered the way people pursue scholarship and research; it has changed the way people use libraries.

Since 1967, OCLC has served libraries and information centers with innovation and dedication. I am honored to take part in celebrating OCLC's 30th anniversary. This article discusses OCLC and the changing Asia Pacific library scene under the broad headings of the three phases of technology innovation. Readers must bear in mind that there are many great libraries with long traditions as well as many modern libraries equipped with advanced technologies in this region. When I refer to libraries in Asia Pacific, I am referring to the majority of libraries in this region, which have not had the resources to make many advances in the past few decades.

ASIA PACIFIC LIBRARIES AND OCLC ASIA PACIFIC SERVICES

Asia Pacific covers a huge space on the globe. The OCLC Asia Pacific Services (APS) services a geographic region that includes China, Japan and Mongolia to the north; Australia and New Zealand to the southeast; and India, Pakistan and Afghanistan to the west. Within these boundaries inhabit 55 percent of the global population. It is a heterogeneous region, consisting of countries both rich and poor, with racial, linguistic and cultural diversity. Fifteen years ago, however, all libraries in Asia, big and small, had one thing in common: there was very little automation in evidence anywhere. Libraries were managed and operated basically as they were decades ago. It was not until the mid-1980s that libraries in this region began to change.

OCLC Asia Pacific Services was established in August 1986. It had grown to 193 users in 1993. Since then, Asia Pacific users have more than tripled: 630 libraries in 12 countries are now using OCLC in 1997. The rapid growth of Asia Pacific OCLC users during this period was a direct result of the global strategy, adopted by the OCLC Board of Trustees and management in June 1993. OCLC established international expansion, expansion of reference services, and enhancement of cataloging and resource sharing services as the three priority areas. This far-sighted strategy not only assured OCLC's lead in technology innovations but also accelerated OCLC's efforts in building a global library network.

In addition to the tireless efforts of the staff of OCLC Asia Pacific

Service, OCLC's partnership with about a dozen local distributors in various countries was also critical to its success in this region. The outstanding examples are Kinokuniya Company in Japan, DA Information Services in Australia and New Zealand, Kyobo Book Center and Orom Computer in South Korea, and Flysheet Information Services in Taiwan. Together they brought OCLC services to more than 600 libraries and institutions. There are now 306 users in Japan, 115 in Korea, 90 in Taiwan, 88 in Australia, 28 in New Zealand, and a growing number of users in Hong Kong, China, India, Malaysia, Singapore, Thailand and the Philippines. One often hears that an excellent product makes an outstanding salesman. It is certainly true in this case.

As stated in OCLC's strategic plan in 1991, paralleling OCLC's expansion were powerful new trends in libraries, in the information industry, in computing and in telecommunications. Jointly, these forces revolutionized library operations and services in the United States. These same forces are now pushing the online revolution in Asia Pacific libraries. Among these forces, advances in telecommunications brought the ability to link networks and to move information at higher speeds. More important, they made OCLC products and services affordable to libraries in the Asia Pacific region.

The economic environment in Asia was also in favor of OCLC's international expansion program. As observed by Andrew Wang, Director of APS, "The Asia Pacific region has experienced one of the world's highest economic growth rates in the past decade. A growing economy increases the need for information. Many of the countries in this region have a rich cultural heritage and many thousand years of history. Economic growth and advancement of technology have created a need for OCLC services."[2]

In 1989, OCLC brought libraries and their users in this region the largest and most comprehensive bibliographic database, WorldCat (the OCLC Online Union Catalog). Along with the WorldCat came Cataloging and Interlibrary Loan Systems. They provide great tools for Asia Pacific libraries to do better today what they did yesterday. In the past ten years, many new products and services have been made available from OCLC to libraries in this region. The three phases of technological innovation seem to have come about for Asia Pacific.

DOING BETTER WHAT WE DID YESTERDAY

Largely due to the scarcity of resources and the lack of overall support in the development of library services, Asian libraries for a long time have faced tough obstacles in making any progress. It is fair to say that in the early 1980s, most of the libraries in Asia compared unfavorably with their counterparts in Europe and North America. With the economic boom of the 1980s, however, many libraries came to realize the importance of delivering accurate and timely products to their constituents. It could not have been a better time for OCLC to explore the Asia market. In 1986, OCLC brought to Asia its years of experience in developing and managing a large bibliographic utility and a shared Cataloging System supporting the input of multilingual scripts. This robust and mature system not only enabled Asian libraries to mechanize many tasks that had been performed manually, but enabled them to do these tasks much better. More important, it provided libraries in this region a much-needed tool to bring their library services up to date, skipping many developmental stages, which libraries in the West have gone through in years, if not decades.

This first phase of change was especially obvious in cataloging efforts. You may remember how cataloging was done in the "pre-bibliographic-utility" days, and even during the early years of shared online cataloging. I can recall vividly the processes I went through when I first implemented the OCLC Cataloging System at SUNY-Buffalo in 1972. The first thing we had to do was to learn the MARC tags and coding. Then we had to work out our card profile including cards for the added and subject entries with the OCLC client representatives. While it was considered a challenge just to ensure that the indicators were properly coded, it was nevertheless a major accomplishment when compared with the time spent in searching the NUC catalog, taking a Polaroid picture of the record, typing the records on cards, and then reproducing the card set. It was only in the early 1980s that libraries in the United States began downloading bibliographic records from OCLC to their local systems. Many libraries in Asia Pacific have been fortunate to be able to bypass these cumbersome steps and to mechanize the manual processes with a highly efficient global network and a huge bibliographic database. Books in Western languages that in the past required a great deal of language and subject expertise can be cataloged with high hit rate and minimum effort today.

Another feature that attracts Asian libraries to OCLC is its large Chinese-Japanese-Korean (CJK) database and its unique CJK software. WorldCat contains about 1.5 million unique CJK records, one of the largest electronic resources of its kind in the world.

CHANGING THE TASKS OF LIBRARIANSHIP

When speaking of Asia Pacific, one cannot overlook China where one quarter of the world's population lives. While many libraries in China engaged in library automation to some degree, they were not very much affected by the computer revolution that was taking place beyond China's borders until August 1996.

August 1996 was not an ordinary month. During this month, WorldCat celebrated its 25th anniversary, and OCLC Asia Pacific Services had its 10th birthday. In addition, OCLC launched a Service Center in China at Tsinghua University on August 27. I consider this event a milestone in the history of librarianship in China. At the dedication ceremony, the president of Tsinghua University said: "It is the desire of Tsinghua University, through this cooperation with OCLC, to enrich network information resources and to modernize the development of library and information services in China." As the site of the China Education and Research Network (CERNET), Tsinghua is best positioned for this mission. Currently, 108 universities are linked on CERNET. It is expected that by the year 2000, the majority of the 1,000 universities and colleges in China will be on CERNET.

What does this event mean to library users? Prof. Daofu Zhang of Shandong University of Technology describes his experience like this: "Using OCLC is faster than riding in a rocket. With it, I am able to travel around the world at the speed of light within a wide span of 4,000 years. OCLC reaches every corner of the world and greatly shortens the distances. It makes the globe magically small and turns a thousand years into an instant by providing the access to any information at the snap of the fingers. OCLC is to me something like an international pass with which I can 'visit' several thousand libraries in more than 100 countries without having to go through the complicated procedures for a passport abroad."[3]

After surfing happily on the Internet and locating exciting information in "every corner of the world," Prof. Zhang will be disappointed if these materials are out of reach. I hope that librarians at Shandong University of Technology will be able to use either the FirstSearch service or OCLC Interlibrary Loan to help Prof. Zhang to acquire the materials.

Resource sharing and interlibrary loan have not been priority programs in Asian libraries. One of the reasons for their limited development has been the lack of accurate holding information and reliable delivery mechanism. In a region where library resources are relatively scarce, cooperation in collection development can play an important part in promoting scholarship and research. When the OCLC Interlibrary Loan Subsystem was activated in 1979, OCLC reengineered the entire ILL process for American libraries. Today, WorldCat is not only the largest database of bibliographic records and of location information in the world, it also supports the most heavily used interlibrary loan system in the world. It is reasonable to expect that with time, OCLC users in the Asia Pacific region will also be able to use the services offered by OCLC to change many traditional library tasks.

TRANSFORMATION OF LIBRARIES
IN THE ASIA PACIFIC REGION

WorldCat and the OCLC shared cataloging system have helped the libraries in the Asia Pacific region to do better today what they did yesterday. These tools and OCLC's expanded resource sharing and interlibrary loan services are changing the tasks of librarianship. I believe FirstSearch with its increasing number of reference and full-text databases, its Electronic Collections Online, and its document delivery program, as well as the state-of-the-art SiteSearch software will help transform many of the Asia Pacific libraries into modern electronic libraries in the not too distant future. I say this because I believe networked information will fill many Asia libraries' fundamental needs in international resources. The situation at *Science* magazine illustrates my point well. According to its editor, *Science*, the largest circulating magazine of its kind, has few subscriptions in China. However, its electronic version will be able to reach scholars in hundreds of Chinese universities later this year.

In June 1997, OCLC launched FirstSearch Electronic Collections Online. In its promotional brochure, it stated that it "is designed to meet the growing needs of libraries in transition from print to electronic serials collection . . . OCLC seeks to reduce your costs for electronic journal access, storage, and contents; enhance your library's role in collection management; and set the stage for integration with the OCLC FirstSearch online reference service." I find this piece of information to be potentially great news to many libraries in this region.

For the more affluent Asia Pacific libraries, such as those in Australia, Hong Kong, Singapore, a large number of electronic resources have been accessible either on their library and campus networks or through the Internet. Libraries in these places choose to use OCLC FirstSearch because it provides an added advantage: a unified user-friendly interface to a large number of databases. Asia Pacific is, however, a region of great diversity. Many of the libraries do not have the means or the foreign currency to acquire Western language materials which they need whether in print or in electronic format. As the need for timely and efficient access to information grows, so does the interest of the less developed Asian libraries in electronic resources. How to empower these Asian libraries to gain access to this information is a challenge for OCLC.

Another OCLC product which seems to have a great potential in assisting the transformation of Asian libraries is SiteSearch software. SiteSearch software allows a library to build, integrate and access Z39.50-based information resources in a World Wide Web environment. It is feasible for libraries in Asia Pacific to organize themselves into convenient groups and to use OCLC SiteSearch software in a way similar to the Georgia Library Learning Online system (GALILEO) or the Committee on Institutional Cooperation (CIC) Virtual Electronic Library project.

When Diebold wrote about the three phases of change brought by innovative technology, he probably did not envision that in certain cases, the lines dividing the three phases would be so blurred that the phases blend into one. I find the introduction of OCLC services in the Asia Pacific region is such a case.

ENRICHING OCLC ONLINE CATALOG WITH ASIAN COLLECTIONS

Being a cataloger at heart, I read with great appreciation the five winning articles on "What the OCLC Online Union Catalog Means to Me." These articles gave excellent examples of the multiple facets of the Online Union Catalog. Patricia L. Hassan's statement, "very proudly I tell you that I have helped to build an international knowledge base," will no doubt be echoed by many catalogers. Hassan went on to write that the "OCLC Union Catalog has endowed new power to the libraries–instead of being 'information archives,' libraries have become 'information access points.' Its impact has been to help launch the global Information Age–in that the scope of information is beyond borders, and cooperation in creating and obtaining that information is a daily, routine affair."[4] I believe all librarians share this view. I would like to discuss how Asia Pacific libraries may participate in building this international knowledge base.

"Institutions in the Asia Pacific region benefit from participation in OCLC cataloging, retrospective conversion, and other services, but it is the entire OCLC community that benefits when bibliographic records from the Asia Pacific region are entered into the OCLC Online Union Catalog," wrote Bob Murphy of OCLC in 1994.[5] After years of negotiation by Andrew Wang, bibliographic records of two significant Asian collections were converted and loaded into WorldCat between 1991 and 1995. These include 32,032 records from the Chinese National Bibliography in the National Library of China and 282,980 Japanese bibliographic records from Waseda University Library. Information on these valuable resources since then have been made available to scholars worldwide.

The OCLC Cataloging System and OCLC CAT CD450 system have been used widely in Asia Pacific. They have pretty much answered all cataloging needs in Western languages for libraries in these countries. But there are few Asian libraries that contribute cataloging records of materials in their own languages into WorldCat. I refer specifically to libraries that catalog Chinese, Japanese, and Korean materials. Chinese and Japanese records combined represent 2.6 percent of the bibliographic records in WorldCat. These two languages are among the ten largest language groups in the union catalog. According to an OCLC CJK statistical report issued on May 23, 1997, only one library out of over 500 OCLC library users in countries or territories where these three languages are used regularly contributes CJK bibliographic records to WorldCat. This means not only cataloging efforts of these libraries cannot be shared by other libraries, but information on their resources cannot be shared either.

While every library must decide for itself what OCLC services to use, I cannot agree more with K. Wayne Smith, when he wrote about "The Tragedy of the Commons" that "Ruin is the destination toward which all men rush, each pursuing his own best interest in a society that believes in freedom of the commons. Freedom in a commons brings ruin to all. In the past 20 years, OCLC member libraries have created a commons that they have used and shared for the benefit of their institutions and their users. That commons is the OCLC Online Union Catalog."[6] Smith went on to state that because of the availability of Internet and various levels of networks, many libraries use OCLC only when they cannot find what they need locally and regionally, which could result in the long run in the demise of WorldCat. While I agree with this observation, I must quickly add that Asian libraries face exceptional obstacles in this regard.

One of my commitments when I came to work in this region in 1990 was to promote CJK applications in libraries. While I have had some success, I also experienced some seemingly insurmountable obstacles. I suspect that these obstacles are universal among Asian libraries when one considers CJK at a "global" level. OCLC has its origin as a bibliographical utility for American libraries, and its CJK system naturally was designed for American libraries. Among Asia Pacific CJK library users, however, there are differences in national MARC formats, character sets, internal codes, cataloging rules, subject headings, classification schemes, authorities and romanization schemes. Beyond these, there are fundamental problems with computer operating systems and CJK enabling software. In the past seven years, I have had discussions about these problems on numerous occasions with various people–librarians, systems vendors, software developers, linguists and researchers in these areas. Invariably, we would conclude that none of us has the power to solve the problems. OCLC can and must help.

On May 21, 1996, the OCLC Users Council unanimously adopted the revised document, "The OCLC Online Union Catalog: Principles of Cooperation." This new version of Principles made one significant change in describing the Online Union Catalog from "national union catalog" to "international union catalog." The document now begins with the sentence that "from its inception, the OCLC Online Union Catalog (OLUC) has been used both as a foundation for shared cataloging and as a *de facto* international union catalog." While the Principles of Cooperation requests that member libraries contribute to OCLC all current bibliographic and holdings information representing cataloged items in their collections, OCLC makes a commitment to facilitate the participation of libraries as authorized users of OCLC records, systems and services.

To facilitate the exchange of CJK records and sharing of resources, OCLC, being the *de facto* international union catalog, has the responsibility to itself and to its users to overcome the technical difficulties that have prevented Asian users from contributing bibliographic records in their native languages. The fact of the matter is that these technical difficulties are interconnected, and no other organization is better positioned to take up the challenges than that of OCLC.

Phyllis Spies, when welcoming guests in March 1995 at the 13th Annual Conference of Research Library Directors (the theme of which was the Global Community of Research Libraries), said: "OCLC's fundamental goals in our international initiatives are to continue to build an international database and to establish a variety of systems and services that will provide the broadest possible access to the world's information for the benefit of scholars and information seekers." Resolving the technical difficulties that prevent Asian libraries from participating fully in the sharing of resources will certainly promote these goals.

Many experts are familiar with our CJK predicaments. The following suggestions may serve as a starting point for discussions and for OCLC to consider. This discussion focuses on topics which will, as the first step, move us toward a more complete international union catalog. It leaves out authorities, classifications schemes, and subject headings. It assumes AACR2 is more or less followed by OCLC users. These suggestions may serve as a catalyst to bringing solutions to the problems of CJK applications.

CJK Character Set: Adopt Unicode

Currently, OCLC, the Library of Congress and RLIN use the East Asia Character Code (EACC). I elaborated some of its problems in 1995.[7]

Today, updating EACC is no longer an option. We must take a further step in adopting Unicode.

It has become obvious that EACC is seldom used outside of libraries. This means vendors have limited incentive for developing enabling software for EACC, and if they do, it is extremely expensive. For example, when we learned that our campus would change to Microsoft Windows 95 in fall 1996, we requested our vendor to update the interface for us early in 1995. To this day, however, our CJK software vendor has not obtained support from Microsoft; therefore, our users must revert to DOS to view our CJK/EACC records. Our Online Public Access Catalog is also available on the World Wide Web, but since our CJK records are in EACC, which is not supported by any Web browsers, users still have problems viewing CJK records.

While Unicode may not answer all of our problems, it seems to offer the best solution, especially if OCLC would lend its support to Unicode by devoting more of its Research and Development efforts to this area.

CJK Enabling Software

Adopting Unicode cannot be achieved overnight, even if OCLC should consider this option. We need interim solutions. As far as we can determine, OCLC is the only organization in the world that has developed CJK/EACC software. OCLC CJK software, an OCLC communications emulation software, is used only for accessing WorldCat. Libraries must equip their local library systems with proper CJK/EACC enabling software so that their patrons can view the EACC records.

OCLC Passport Software (English version) has incorporated Telnet access to a library's own catalog. It would be a great service if OCLC could enhance the CJK software and make the same feature available to CJK users. In addition to a Telnet solution, a Web browser enabling program would be most welcome as well. Perhaps Java technology may help in this regard.

Recently, I have read with interest about the OCLC CJK Public Access Pilot Project on the Web and am looking forward to seeing follow-up development continue.

Allow Multi-Bibliographic Formats

OCLC supports only USMARC format in inputting and outputting from WorldCat. It seems feasible for OCLC to enhance its Cataloging interface and the CJK software to allow more flexibility for libraries to upload and download CJK records in other formats, such as Chinese-MARC, CN-MARC and Japan-MARC. This is, however, only the first step.

Using USMARC to catalog CJK materials, catalogers must create parallel 880 fields for vernacular characters, a cumbersome and time-consuming procedure. In libraries in China, Japan and Korea, catalog records consist of vernacular characters without romanization; thus, 880 fields are not used. These records, therefore, do not meet OCLC standards and cannot be entered into WorldCat. This is an undesirable situation for both OCLC and other OCLC users. OCLC could develop a mechanism to either provide romanization of each field on the fly or to allow these records to reside in WorldCat at a specifically designated level.

In fact, some progress has been made in this respect. The integrated library system installed in many university libraries in Hong Kong and in the National Library of Australia can provide Chinese romanization automatically in bibliographic records. This software greatly reduces the keying required when cataloging Chinese materials. Catalogers simply enter the Chinese characters into the appropriate fields in the record, and the system automatically converts Chinese characters into their romanized forms and places the vernacular script in the equivalent 880 fields of the MARC record. A similar capability in the Cataloging System will enable OCLC to take in catalog records created by many libraries in Asia Pacific and further enrich WorldCat to the benefit of its users.

A more drastic but fundamental step to take in this regard would be to adopt SGML or any similar scheme in the long run.

Pinyin versus Wade-Giles for Chinese Records

Pinyin versus Wade-Giles has been an over-debated topic among East Asian libraries in the United States. It is, however, a nonissue for libraries where Chinese is the spoken language since romanization in general is not necessary.

There are complicated issues involved in making a change. This issue has already dragged on too long; OCLC perhaps should take a position in this debate and engage itself in helping libraries to resolve these issues.

In the March/April 1995 issue of the *OCLC Newsletter,* Smith wrote that "the OCLC Board of Trustees approved a new international business plan that calls for OCLC to make significant new investments in its international systems, products, people, and services." He went on to report that over the next five years, OCLC will, among other initiatives:

- Enhance its database loading software to permit loading of UNI-MARC in order to more easily enrich WorldCat with international titles
- Enhance the CJK system to support international standards and more transliteration schemes
- Develop interfaces for FirstSearch

My suggestions are not much more than what OCLC promised in 1995.

"JOURNEY TO THE 21ST CENTURY"

"In the next phase of the online revolution, libraries are expected to actively provide information to users in the form they want, when and where they need it. This journey to the 21st century promises to be an exciting, challenging, and ultimately, rewarding voyage to the new frontiers of information service."[8] These words expressed by OCLC in 1991 are still valid today. I expect that libraries in the Asia Pacific region will become valued partners of OCLC beyond 2000.

NOTES

1. Smith, K. Wayne. 1993. "OCLC: Changing the Tasks of Librarianship," *Library Hi Tech* (November): 7.

2. Wang, Andrew. 1995. "Connecting the East and the West: A Case Study," *The Global Community of Research Libraries: Proceedings of the Thirteenth Annual Conference of Research Library Directors.*

3. Zhang, Daofu. 1996. "What the OCLC Online Union Catalog Means to Me." *OCLC Newsletter* (July/August), No. 222: 31.

4. Hassan, Patricia L. 1996. "What the OCLC Online Union Catalog Means to Me." *OCLC Newsletter* (July/August), No. 222: 29.

5. Murphy, Bob. 1994. "Availability of Asian Records Helps Libraries Worldwide." *OCLC Newsletter* (March/April) No. 208: 15.

6. Smith, K. Wayne. 1993. "OCLC: Changing the Tasks of Librarianship," *Library Hi Tech* (November):15.

7. Chang, Min-min. 1995. "Far Away, But Next Door," *The Global Community of Research Libraries: Proceedings of the Thirteenth Annual Conference of Research Library Directors.*

8. OCLC. 1991. "Journey to the 21st Century: OCLC's Strategic Plan."

OCLC in Europe

Christine Deschamps

Once upon a time there was a wonderful tale of the OCLC . . . After Cinderella became a princess, she had children in other countries. And that is how OCLC came to be born in Europe! Once again, the United States was bearing blessings from across the Atlantic. And yet, it was not that easy. . . .

After all, Frederick G. Kilgour, the founder of OCLC, did in fact write in 1974: "At that time [when it was created in 1967], there was no similar organization in the United States, and no one thought it would really work . . . What then would be said in Europe?"

THE EARLY DAYS

David Buckle, the first Director of OCLC Europe, remembers hearing about the work of Kilgour and the Ohio College Library Center (OCLC) throughout the 1970s. He met Kilgour briefly for the first time in October 1978 at a conference in Trondheim, Norway. Kilgour had already succeeded in achieving outstanding cooperation among American librarians, in both the technological and operational areas. Buckle was pursuing the same goal in Birmingham: the standardized application of computer technology to the daily operations of libraries, with interlibrary cooperation.

Christine Deschamps is Director, Université René Descartes, Paris V Library.

The author wishes to thank Phyllis B. Spies, Janet Mitchell, and especially David Buckle, for their assistance and generous gift of their time in the preparation of this article.

[Haworth co-indexing entry note]: "OCLC in Europe." Deschamps, Christine. Co-published simultaneously in *Journal of Library Administration* (The Haworth Press, Inc.) Vol. 25, No. 2/3, 1998, pp. 141-157; and: *OCLC 1967-1997: Thirty Years of Furthering Access to the World's Information* (ed: K. Wayne Smith) The Haworth Press, Inc., 1998, pp. 141-157. Single or multiple copies of this article are available for a fee from The Haworth Document Delivery Service [1-800-342-9678, 9:00 a.m. - 5:00 p.m. (EST). E-mail address: getinfo@haworthpressinc.com].

At the same time, other projects were also emerging in Europe, especially in Scandinavia, the United Kingdom, the Netherlands, Germany, Belgium and Italy. Most were publicly funded projects. At the time, Buckle had been responsible since 1970 for computerizing the University of Birmingham library, which quite naturally formed part of the "BLCMP" (Birmingham Libraries Co-operative Mechanization Project). This project was launched in 1969 and received government grants to develop and introduce a shared computerized cataloging system, and thus create a collective catalog, initially of the three founding members (Aston University and the public libraries of the City of Birmingham, in addition to the University of Birmingham). In 1971, he became director of BLCMP and in 1977, CEO of the company "BLCMP Library Services," which was converted into a nonprofit corporation.

Kilgour was not only an author extremely dedicated to the cause of libraries, but also a very popular speaker capable of holding an audience's attention. His presentations were very convincing. His style with Europeans was something akin to a colonial preacher, with a total conviction that his message would bring the good word to everyone.

This conference in Trondheim, Norway, brought together the heads of all major library automation projects in Europe, to discuss current and future developments. Many of these projects were already operational and some were based on the use of new products. They clearly had reached a turning point: they were emerging from the publicly funded research phase and finding themselves faced with the hard reality of a commercial future. OCLC had already passed this stage, so we could learn a lot from its experience.

At the time, in the UK, five major library automation projects had received public funding: the Library Services Division of the British Library, BLCMP, SWALCAP (South West Academic Libraries Co-operative Automation Project), LASER (London and South Eastern Region library bureau) and SCOLCAP (Scottish Libraries Co-operative Automation Project). By 1978, most had already completed their development programs and were seeking other, more commercial sources of funding. They therefore formed a loose-knit cooperative group known as CAG (Co-operative Automation Group), with the idea of studying the feasibility of creating a collective national catalog that would form the core of a national network, roughly imitating that developed in the United States with OCLC. These plans were never carried out, however.

The meeting in Trondheim gave Kilgour the opportunity to speak directly with the directors of interlibrary cooperative networks and to learn about their achievements and aspirations. In turn, these directors were pleased to learn about the structure and organization of OCLC and study how it originated from the Ohio university and college library community to serve a national community of university, college, research, regional, public and specialized libraries through regional and national networks. Kilgour found this a unique chance to build on the opportunities and challenges that Europe could provide for his dream of expanding OCLC beyond the United States, to the various nations in the Old World.

Quite obviously, Kilgour then decided that it was worth committing more of his time and OCLC funds to Europe. He retained Butler Cox, a consulting firm, to conduct a feasibility study.

This study was to address two serious problems in all the major European countries: the status and regulation of telecommunications infrastructures, as well as the state of library science and its computer development.

At the same time, Kilgour instituted a policy of meeting with the heads of most national, university, college, research and public libraries in the UK. He also consulted the heads of cooperative library networks to begin a dialog on cooperation with OCLC. This is how Buckle and Kilgour came to know each other so well.

By early 1980, Kilgour had concluded that Europe merited his commitment and that the UK was definitely the most promising site in Europe for establishing the OCLC bridgehead, given the shared language, culture and library tradition. All he needed was a partner.

With this in mind, Kilgour met with virtually all networks in the fall of 1980, and a contract ultimately was signed with BLCMP, which became the OCLC service center in the United Kingdom. At that time, he believed this shared cataloging system, which had prospered so well among librarians in the United States, should perform just as well in Europe, requiring no investment in any change whatsoever to allow for the specific needs or special traditions of each group of librarians in Europe.

Thus, the first OCLC international service center was to be installed in England to continue and coordinate the work of European network centers, and to house the transatlantic communications hub and the connection with European telecommunications systems. This office opened in January 1981 under the direction of Buckle. In December 1980, however, the OCLC Board of Trustees appointed a new President, Rowland C.W. Brown, to replace Kilgour, who had announced in March 1980 that he was stepping down from day-to-day management of OCLC. OCLC would take a year to reconsider its international adventure.

This hiatus was both good and bad for OCLC in Europe. European librarians interpreted it as hesitancy, and the contract governing networking agreements with BLCMP was never executed. The OCLC Board of

Trustees had reason to be cautious, and was seeking to identify more clearly the costs and benefits of this initiative. Brown developed a strategic plan for OCLC in Europe, which the Board approved in November 1981. This strategic plan identified the market potential presented by the UK, as well as the type of investment required. It also analyzed conditions in the UK market.

However, in the 12 months between the new president's arrival and the Board's approval of the strategic plan, much water had gone under the bridge for OCLC in Europe. The enthusiasm and expectations of 1979 and 1980 had been eclipsed by growing hostility toward what was now considered a direct threat to library automation companies in Europe. This trend was especially strong in the UK, where OCLC had decided to open its first office, and OCLC made a brave response.

It must be clearly understood that during the same 12 months following approval of the strategic plan, OCLC had created the necessary infrastructure to market the online shared cataloging service. This initiative required great energy and creativity, as it had to create a national telecommunications network to link the regional nodes. The European regional node was located in Birmingham, in the offices of OCLC Europe, which also served as the terminal for the transatlantic line from Dublin, Ohio. There were regional nodes in Scotland, Ireland, Wales and the rest of England. Unlike the United States, most European librarians wanted more from computer cataloging applications than just index cards. They wanted COM microfiches as well. Yet in 1982, OCLC was offering only cards.

In association with an independent firm, LIBPAC, OCLC Europe developed a system to manage a collective regional catalog, from which subsets updated twice weekly could be extracted in special formatting to have COM microfiches produced locally by computer and microcopy service providers.

It obviously is difficult from the outset to penetrate a foreign market already well served by national suppliers, including the country's national library. But when a company also shows hesitancy and a lack of genuine support for investing in adaptations to the existing market, this is not likely to inspire confidence. OCLC's rivals, especially the national library networks, naturally chose to capitalize on this difficult situation. The British Library, for example, first decided not to grant OCLC a license to access the British National Bibliography, a necessary step for anyone wanting to promote a shared cataloging service to the library community in the UK.

Ever innovative, OCLC Europe marshaled the cooperation of British publishers, who sent the offices of OCLC Europe a copy of the title pages of their new publications, and a team of catalogers worked on directly entering the data into the OCLC online collective catalog.

OCLC Europe's inventiveness, however, could not overcome a major handicap to marketing a viable shared cataloging product: limited hours of access. In 1982, when OCLC Europe was ready to provide a competitive product to the UK, its system was only available from 8:00 a.m. to 8:00 p.m., United States Eastern Time. As a result, it was not available in England before 1:00 p.m., and in the rest of Europe, before 2:00 p.m. Only when the new OCLC Online System was introduced in the early 1990s did European libraries begin to enjoy the same hours of access as their American counterparts. Other difficulties persisted, and these will be examined later.

From the beginning, Kilgour, however, believed that these difficulties apparently mattered little compared with the wealth of the online collective catalog provided by OCLC. All providers of services to libraries realize that their users seek the most exhaustive services available in the library field. That is also why Kilgour decided in 1967 to shift from offline to online mode. He had a gift for making demonstrations look like magic. While he served as master of ceremonies, his wife Eleanor performed miracles on her terminal. These demonstrations won over "converts." There was no mention of "buying" or "selling," but prospects were charmed. At a time when everyone is used to surfing the Internet, it is hard to realize how impressive an online demonstration could be, using a database located 6,000 kilometers across the Atlantic Ocean.

Like all magic tricks, these long-distance demonstrations demanded meticulous planning, yet despite the best-laid plans, something always went wrong. Some demonstration sites dated back to the Middle Ages, but most usually suffered from 19th century technology. Buckle remembered one of the first OCLC terminal models, the Beehive, a cumbersome metal box. (Note: It was never intended to be portable.) In particular, he had to conduct a demonstration in the office of the curator of a prestigious university. This office was located in a 13th century monastery where he had to carry the Beehive terminal and acoustic modem up a narrow spiral stone staircase. When he had finally set his equipment down and mopped his brow, he prepared to connect it to the telephone. But he was handed a bakelite antique which obviously was incompatible with an acoustic modem. This was when he realized that it was not enough to ask in advance, "Do you have a telephone in your office with a direct line?" He had to trundle all his equipment back down the stairs. But, once it was connected in the cataloger's office, he could work his magic and win over new converts.

By the mid-1980s, OCLC was well established in Europe. It was now time to venture into other countries on the continent. In 1985, a new master plan was developed for Europe and approved by the OCLC Board. This plan studied the installation of OCLC on the European continent, following many meetings and seminars organized with the heads of major libraries in northwestern Europe. Brown played a key role at these meetings, as he was very familiar with European habits after working many years on the continent. He had even studied in Paris as a youth, and this would prove very useful.

FROM EARLY PROMISE TO HARD-WON RESULTS . . .

In 1985, at the meeting of the Association of Research Libraries at Rice University, Houston, Texas, the president of the university, Dr. Sam Carrington, met with both Brown and Denis Varloot, then Director, Libraries, Museums, and Scientific and Technical Information Branch (DBMIST), responsible for French university libraries, who had become a close and highly esteemed friend of Dr. Carrington's. This meeting was the first in a long series and marked the start of negotiations between OCLC and France. It should be noted that unlike arrangements in other countries, OCLC in Dublin, Ohio, had always been very closely involved in the French agreements, although OCLC Europe was still present.

The first official meeting in Paris was chaired by Dr. Carrington. These negotiations came at the right time: like the UK, France was devoid of shared computerized cataloging networks and was beginning to feel a pressing need for this tool. OCLC also saw a major market with long-term prospects for growth opening up at a time when it was sidelined in the UK. A shared interest therefore presided over the negotiations, certainly the best condition for a favorable outcome.

Brown's experience in the French business world made him the best possible person to lead these negotiations. Across the table, he would find in Varloot the same level of technical knowledge, the same willingness to stake his reputation on this venture, and long-term vision of the potential benefits for the librarian community. Together, they got the ball rolling: in 1981, only one library had signed an agreement with OCLC Europe; by 1985, there were about 40.

As the negotiations with France progressed, the British Library finally realized the potential offered by OCLC and opened up its database. Until then, it had participated solely in OCLC's interlibrary lending system, by providing its locations to the British Library Lending Division (BLLD). This time, the scope was broader: the Library Services Division approved the purchase and download of entries in UKMARC format. At the same time, Brian Perry, Director, Department of Research and Development, British Library, became the first non-U.S. member of the OCLC Research and Development Advisory Committee. Perry helped forge links with Sir Peter Swinnerton-Dyer, president of the University Grant Committee and a member of the Higher Education Committee. This scientific recognition of the abilities and potential role of OCLC was strengthened by the trips Brown made during this time in Europe to all the largest libraries, striving to establish contacts with Germany (especially the brand new Deutsches BibliotheksInstitut), France, Scandinavia (with university community cooperative groups) and the Netherlands (with PICA).

The various retrospective conversion operations also began at this time, and marked the real turning point in the growth of OCLC in Europe. OCLC also began proposing extensions to the cataloging system, for accessions, control of periodicals, and a series of integrated accounting and statistical services.

Around 1980, OCLC had begun distributing the LS 2000 local library system (the first in Europe was installed at the Newcastle Library). But this came to the European market too late and the price to be paid was very heavy. It proved a total failure, and the Newcastle Library was also the first to stop using LS 2000.

Retrospective conversion also had trouble starting up. OCLC wanted operations to be conducted in the United States, but the European libraries strongly resisted the idea of sending files abroad (reliable, fast transportation was not as readily available as it is today). Yet the market was huge! In Birmingham, there were as many as 25 people working on this task at the same time, just for European libraries.

SERIOUS RESTRUCTURING

In 1989, the arrival of Dr. K. Wayne Smith as OCLC's third president and CEO was marked by extensive reorganization and restructuring. Retrospective conversion for European libraries would no longer be done in the UK, but in Dublin, Ohio, and the Birmingham team shrank from 36 to 12. Psychologically, it was hard to make such a drastic cut while continuing business development. But with hindsight, there is no doubt that this move was necessary. While Brown was an excellent executive with a solid grasp of the requirements of an international venture, his vision may have been too broad, too "scattered."

Smith began to tighten up OCLC's approach in Europe by refocusing on what would actually make money in the medium and long term. He believed that the international operation was becoming part of OCLC's culture. OCLC Europe was no longer an appendage that occasionally proved bothersome. The international venture was finally accepted as a tool for growth and was managed accordingly. It was becoming an integral part of daily operations in Dublin, Ohio. Everything was revisited from this new perspective. In a specific example, retrospective conversion clearly was no longer considered just a separate service; it finally enjoyed recognition as an important component for growth and enrichment of WorldCat (the OCLC Online Union Catalog), OCLC's major tool and prime asset.

Cooperation with France became solidly established, particularly through major retrospective conversion agreements, which led to special financial agreements, called "marchés" in French legal terminology. These agreements, mandatory for any transaction exceeding 300,000 FF, are covered by specific schedules of technical specifications (CCTP) and administrative clauses (CCAP), are reviewed by a special commission on information services contracts (CSMI), and finally, must be signed by the Financial Comptroller, an official delegated to each ministry by the Ministry of the Budget, who is totally independent and occasionally takes his time to sign major agreements involving several million francs. Buckle remembers long and arduous negotiations during which France's Ministry of National Education tried to explain the ministry's procedures, the mandatory administrative wording of the documents, and the time required. In turn, he had to explain to OCLC the reasons for the delays in start-up, and had to ask them to trust in the French system without knowing it. The author is sure Buckle developed some premature gray hair during this period. The agreements were eventually signed, and the collective catalog for French university libraries to date contains almost 2,000,000 entries from OCLC WorldCat, almost two thirds of the total.

Expansion of contacts to Central Europe and Russia began in the early 1990s. The 57th IFLA Conference held in Moscow in 1991 brought the first contacts, despite the turmoil of political events. Then in 1993-1994, the first contacts were made with Slovakia, Hungary, Slovenia, the Czech Republic and Croatia, followed by Poland in 1995. The trying financial circumstances in these countries at first allowed only one-way agreements: they exchanged their national libraries for payment in hard cash (dollars!). This was followed by a strategic plan to expand the field of operations.

Starting in 1995, OCLC Europe began making initial contacts in Africa and parts of Asia, but only the richest and most developed countries in these regions could truly participate: Israel, a few countries in the Middle East, and South Africa.

HOW TO START WORKING WITH OCLC

We find that with the exception of France, most countries have come to OCLC gradually, one library at a time, and one type of operation at a time. The very first library in Europe to use OCLC was the Center for Technical Research in Finland, which began using the OCLC interlibrary loan system before the offices of OCLC Europe were opened. (The first two universities to use the cataloging services in 1982 were the Universities of Essex and Newcastle.)

In England, the British Library Lending Division at Boston Spa also began with interlibrary loans, first as a supplier, then gradually as a full user for requests sent to the United States. It continues to use OCLC to search locations throughout the world.

In 1983, the Edinburgh University Library launched a major seven-year retrospective conversion program. Then in 1985, entries in UK MARC format created by the British Library were added to the OCLC database following an agreement reached by the British Library and OCLC.

In 1986, this gradual approach was enabling OCLC to work with libraries in the UK, Belgium, Denmark, Finland, the Republic of Ireland and Switzerland. This gradual approach was the rule, except in France. In fact, as we have already noted, the negotiations in France had started initially for a specific group, university libraries. After taking part in the initial tests, the National Library had pulled back, as had the Books and Reading Branch for public libraries. Without delay, the agreements were discussed by the Ministry of National Education and OCLC, for cataloging in the library community. This approach heralded the eventual membership of 42 libraries in 1996 (compared with four in 1987!). On the other hand, it is noteworthy that not all French libraries participate in interlibrary lending, and there are still very few that actually use it.

In the other European countries, however, OCLC used a broader range of approaches: ILL, cataloging, retrospective conversion, bibliographic research in reference services. In 1986, the German Libraries Institute signed an agreement for a test with seven German research libraries that would allow certain American OCLC libraries to query the collective catalogs of periodicals and monographs developed by the Deutsches BibliotheksInstitut: the "Zeitschriftendatenbank," produced by the State Library of the Prussian Cultural Foundation, and the DBI Verbundkatalog, containing an authorities file with 250,000 entries. In Spain, cooperation led to the use of interlibrary lending, especially at the University of Barcelona in Catalonia.

National libraries also had a special role to play in OCLC international expansion. In North America, the Library of Congress and the National

Library of Canada had already given the growth of OCLC a solid boost through their cooperation agreements. In Europe, these national libraries had also chosen the OCLC cataloging system: the British Library, National Library of Scotland and National Library of Wales. Since 1990, the opening of Central Europe and Russia has led to work with the National Libraries of the Czech Republic, Slovenia, Hungary and Russia. The work on UNIMARC played an important role in negotiations with these national libraries.

Sometimes, requests came from libraries that had suffered major disasters or damage. For example, the University Library in Metz, France, requested an extremely important retrospective conversion operation following a flood in 1986 that destroyed the catalog as well as a large part of the collection. It had received donations, but without matching cards, no one could now determine which works were actually in the Library in either the old or the new collection.

There was the even more dramatic case of the National Library of Bosnia. Totally destroyed in the recent war in Yugoslavia, the library first wanted to reconstitute its catalog of Bosniaca before rebuilding the library and buying back or recovering books. It would be a new virtual library if ever there was one, a library that only OCLC could retrieve from the void into which it had been plunged by this absurd and barbaric war. WorldCat contains 104,000 entries of Bosniaca and these will restore the collections with those works or reproductions on microfiche or digital support. Although it will be impossible to buy back all the books, this catalog will enable researchers to locate the documents they require and obtain them through interlibrary loan, even before the first book has been returned to its place in the stacks.

Sometimes, it is the need for an interlibrary loan system that creates the link between a European library and OCLC. Very few countries have created their own national interlibrary lending system capable of rivaling the OCLC system. Even less common, if not totally non-existent, is a European interlibrary lending system capable of querying a library data bank of 37 million entries, with locations regularly updated, despite the current problems of postal delays. We have also seen that UK libraries began working through the British Library Lending Division (which later became the British Library Document Supply Centre) in 1981, with a special preferred user status. In 1986, the Statsbibliotek in Arhus began to access the OCLC lending subsystem. In Finland, the Center for Technical Research has used ILL since 1980, and in 1986 it was adopted by the Technological University of Helsinki.

In 1992, OCLC signed an agreement with CURL (Consortium of University Research Libraries) that allows participating libraries to use OCLC for their cataloging and for retrospective conversion. The entries from these libraries were loaded into the WorldCat database.

It was during this period that a new OCLC approach was created: FirstSearch provided access to the bibliographic information not only in the OCLC database, but also from searches of other large bibliographic data banks (MEDLINE, Chemical Abstracts Service, ABI/INFORM, or others), not just for professionals (through the EPIC service), but also for the end user, unfamiliar with these types of queries. The first European libraries to use FirstSearch in 1994 were the Cambridge University Library, Glasgow University Library and the Oxford Library. FirstSearch was available in England through the NISS gateway, under an agreement with CHEST (Combined Higher Education Software Team), an organization whose purpose is to serve as a forum for negotiations between suppliers and the UK community of institutions of higher education and research. WorldCat, ArticleFirst and ContentsFirst were among the most popular bases, especially since the British Library database had entered its titles in ArticleFirst and ContentsFirst. FirstSearch suddenly became a considerable aid for English libraries that encountered difficulty surveying their collections.

Also in 1994, PICA (the Netherlands foundation for cooperation between university libraries and the Royal Netherlands Library) became the first group of libraries in Europe to use OCLC SiteSearch software to access FirstSearch through PICA's own Z39.50 software. Five Dutch university libraries took part in this test. That same year, European libraries could use the services of "distributors" marketing OCLC products, without entering into a direct relationship with OCLC Europe. In France, DOC & Co. is working in conjunction with AUROC, and the market is shared on very clear terms that do not automatically rule out cooperation whenever this is desirable for French libraries.

In 1995, the bloc of countries from the former Soviet Union and Central Europe began to join OCLC. Czechoslovakia, Hungary, Romania, Latvia and Russia that year began retrospective conversion operations or cataloging agreements, often starting with tests. The Russian National Library for Science and Technology began with a three-month test of OCLC Cataloging and Resource Sharing, to master the techniques and train staff. Similarly, the organization of an ongoing seminar entitled "New Information Technology Outlook" was conducted throughout Russia for one month.

The Institute for Information Science (IZUM) signed an agreement with OCLC to open FirstSearch to libraries in Slovenia, using the Z39.50 Access option so libraries can use their local systems to query the First-

Search bibliographic data bases. Thus, IZUM was able to provide all libraries in the country–even very small ones–with end-user access to all the wealth of information contained in FirstSearch, but through interfaces familiar to users, and in their own language. Even further afield, beyond Eastern Europe, contacts were made in 1996 with libraries in Israel, South Africa and Azerbaijan.

Finally, the author must point out the extent to which emergence of the Internet has played an important role in the growth of OCLC in Europe, the Near East and Africa.

PROBLEMS FACING EUROPEAN LIBRARIES USING OCLC

The main drawback for the poorest libraries in European countries is quite clearly the cost: although OCLC is a nonprofit organization (a fact little known outside the United States), its charges must reflect not only the cost of operations, but also the investment in ongoing development of new products and services. The charges seem even higher since they do not cover purchase of a local library management system (as in the case of the SIBIL system in France and Switzerland, for example). Of course, OCLC refunds a certain amount (which has actually exceeded three million francs for French libraries since the start of agreements with OCLC), in the form of cataloging and resource sharing credits, but some countries still find it difficult to afford OCLC. This is often the objection raised when services are promoted in Eastern Europe or Russia, for example, and there is no doubt that without patronage or major public funding, OCLC remains an unattainable dream for some countries. It often proves difficult to draw the fine line between the profits needed for ongoing business development, and an investment that may lose money initially, but prove profitable in the end. OCLC already applies a very generous policy of free test and trial periods to "hook" clients. This situation often proves to be a true torment of Tantalus for some small libraries. It would be interesting if OCLC could establish a clear international investment policy, drawing some funds from other large organizations: IFLA, UNESCO, Soros Foundation, Mellon Foundation, etc.

A second major difficulty for some European countries is the adoption of a different bibliographic format. Changing to USMARC is by no means easy, although OCLC fortunately is now prepared to provide its entries in UNIMARC, and is participating in the work of the IFLA UNIMARC Committee. Nonetheless, there are still problems for two reasons. First, some countries have resolutely insisted on keeping their local format. German libraries are just beginning to agree to abandon the MABI format, under the REUSE project, and following their example, Russian libraries are working on a project to produce descriptions of bibliographic documents and create a compatible RUSSMARC format. In any event, the transition from a national format to an international format always poses a problem. Catalogers must agree to change their habits, and resistance to change is often strong in European libraries. And, they must take appropriate training that is expensive to set up. Second, cataloging is not just a question of computer bibliographic format, it is also a set of work rules. Here again, catalogers must forsake old habits and take training. Abandoning RAK (German alphabetical cataloging rules), let alone the old Prussian rules still used in a few libraries, to use AACR2 represents a full-blown cultural revolution that is not easily instituted. The inevitable lapses into old cataloging methods often lead to inconsistency in the reporting of secondary entries or in errors that are difficult to locate or correct.

Another major problem arises from the diversity of languages spoken in Europe besides English. Here again, the problems vary in nature. In the bibliographic database, under the author or subject headings, it is difficult to adopt the terms recommended by American authority files. When OCLC cataloging and the internal consistency of Library of Congress authority files are implemented in a country such as France where other collective national catalogs are being produced at the same time, radical choices must be made if the goal is to be understood by users consulting OPACs who do not read English. National collective catalogs must also be consistent, and this further complicates the situation.

For author headings, consideration must also be given (in Russian or Greek, for example) to the fact that transliteration based on English phonetics is not necessarily comprehensible in these two countries, or even in others accustomed to their own national transliteration protocol. Chekov in English, for example, may become Tchékov in French, Tschekow in German, etc.

The problem is even more serious for subject headings: Library of Congress subject headings (LCSH) must actually be translated. This was done in France using the Quebec/Canadian translation known as "Répertoire Matières Laval," through the RAMEAU lexical data bank, better adapted to French customs and common terminology. Not all countries are prepared to use a single English subject index system, and the collation and note areas must also be translated.

Similarly, on a practical level, the problem of character sets is a serious issue for many European countries: many want to include in their entries diacritical signs that do not exist in the English entry to be derived. The problem has been temporarily resolved with the pending adoption of the

UNICODE standard. But as OCLC reaches more agreements with a growing number of countries, it must increasingly cope with this type of problem!

Finally, the last problem, which is now close to being solved, is hours of access to the system. Fortunately, WorldCat is now accessible almost 24 hours a day, although connecting to OCLC on the Internet after 3:00 p.m. in Europe is not easy, and response times occasionally can be very slow. When will there be a mirror site in Europe? We should remember as well that Central and Eastern European countries (Russia and the former Soviet republics) still lack good connections–or any connections–to the Internet. The Soros Foundation has given Russia several billion dollars to create an Internet network, but much remains to be done.

BENEFITS OF USING OCLC

The above remarks on the difficulties and problems encountered in participating in OCLC should not mislead European librarians: I am thoroughly convinced that the benefits of using OCLC infinitely outweigh the problems described above, which are all now being solved in any event. There are many benefits.

First and foremost, there is the quality and size of the WorldCat database. With more than 37 million entries from around the world and with a growth rate of one new entry every 15 seconds, it is an incomparable tool. For cataloging, bibliographic identification, document location, and a scientific accessions and collection development policy, no equivalent can be found anywhere else. This unique resource, the result of work by librarians the world over, facilitates knowledge and increases the visibility of various cultures and specialized collections that were previously little known. The consistency of cataloging (authority files), standardization of access, speed of response time, the quality of entries with a systematic entry enrichment policy (in particular with a very complete title), constant updating, the flexibility of parameters which allows the addition of local data to any downloaded entry (including, for example, the addition of subject headings translated from English into the national language) all make WorldCat a unique tool and all the libraries using it recognize this. It contains entries not found anywhere else, dating back further in time than most bibliographic databases, thanks to retrospective conversion operations. The diversity of media, fields, languages and cultures represented is extraordinary and clearly makes WorldCat the jewel of OCLC, both for OCLC itself and for member libraries.

Membership in OCLC means not only making the most of its outstanding potential but also participating directly as a player, and joining the international community of librarians (63 countries, 25,000 libraries). OCLC has national user groups (AUROC in France), working groups by library type, the OCLC Users Council (to which OCLC Europe sends a representative) and has now opened its Board of Trustees to international representatives. The collegial approach is well established, and the documentation sent to libraries (although in English only) is complete and detailed.

But OCLC is more than just cataloging. A growing range of related products is offered concurrently to European libraries. The most important clearly are FirstSearch, Interlibrary Loan (ILL), the Dewey Decimal Classification, retrospective conversion operations separate from current cataloging, and FirstSearch Electronic Collections Online.

Queries by FirstSearch and SiteSearch of the main bibliographic data banks and WorldCat produce an outstanding set of bibliographic data. Linked to SiteSearch and using connection methods based on the Z39.50 standard for client-server architectures, searches are remarkably effective. Users can query the catalogs of large libraries and their own Internet catalog, and in fact, no bibliographic citation can now truly elude library users.

The location of entries, regularly updated on WorldCat, provides a high-performance interlibrary loan system. European libraries can now order photocopies or documents from American libraries, and in particular can publicize and enhance their own collections. Some French libraries have seen loan requests from the United States double or even triple since their locations were incorporated into the base.

Of course, publication of the Dewey Decimal Classification is also a major asset for OCLC and French-language European libraries, since the DDC was translated into French by ASTED. If all libraries in the world used the same classification method, it would be much easier to survey collections.

Retrospective conversion is a major OCLC asset in Europe. In fact, European libraries have few other options: it is very expensive to have a service company capture entries by the thousands, and only OCLC provides this service (in France, for example, university libraries retrospectively converted more than one million entries).

Finally, the emergence in Europe of the electronic document will focus very specifically on the electronic products provided by OCLC: electronic reviews, archiving and storage, access. OCLC can accommodate all of these. For telecommunications, we could mention the example of cooperation between OCLC Europe and France, by which the OCLC subsidiary

"ID France" provides technical assistance to French libraries experiencing difficulties in this area. In the future, OCLC must continue to develop greater awareness of the problems specific to European libraries. In many universities, players are widely dispersed. Universities often have research centers dependent on various authorities (Ministry of Higher Education, Research or Health, National Centers of Scientific Research, etc.). Institutions are not all grouped on a large campus as in the United States. On the contrary, due to local constraints (old cities), we find a large geographic dispersal of institutions, which produces different working conditions from those in the United States. Finally, rigid administrative procedures, the small number of documents compared with the United States, and linguistic plurality could defeat OCLC if it does not give these circumstances adequate consideration.

In general, OCLC is not content merely to offer its products: it is taking charge of support for libraries, developing a realistic timeline for them and providing the necessary training and documentation. When French libraries needed an extension of deadlines for transition from one cataloging medium to another (CAT CD450 in DOS to online cataloging in Windows), they obtained specific timeline changes that allowed them to plan a smooth transition to the new products, and an optimal choice of the various new options. This is one of the great advantages of OCLC: it is designed to provide libraries with the services they request and need. This is a vast difference from (although not a criticism of) certain national bibliographic agencies that may sell entries at a lower cost, but show little concern for the impact on user libraries when, for example, they decide to change format (this concern is not their responsibility!). On the other hand, OCLC provides support to libraries, negotiates discounts on the purchase of computer hardware, assists with the introduction of networks, facilitates telecom access, and allows European libraries to move gradually from a condition that in some cases is closer to the 19th than the 20th century, to the advanced technology of the 21st century. Even the smallest libraries can benefit: we have already mentioned the fact that the option of Z39.50 access to FirstSearch lets libraries in Slovenia use their local systems to query the FirstSearch bibliographic databases, thereby giving their users access to a wealth of information through familiar interfaces, in their own language. No other document supplier can provide this today.

CONCLUSION

Despite the diversity of national situations, OCLC is now widely used in Europe. Massive introduction of the Internet as well as changes in products, the variety of which is highly appreciated, show that the use of services in Europe may be more advanced in research and new technologies than developments in the USA. Arriving later in an information world where cataloging is no longer the only game in town, European countries are taking a different approach to OCLC resources. It is still to be hoped that increasingly closer relations will develop between European and American users, as they work together toward universal access.

BIBLIOGRAPHY

AGOSTINI, Francis, and Catherine LUPOVICI. 1977. *Coopération et réseaux de bibliothéques aux Etats-Unis*. Villeurbanne: ENSSIB.

KILGOUR, F.G. 1974. "Premiers pas vers une nouvelle bibliothéconomie: Ohio College Library Center." *Bulletin des Bibliothéques de France*. 19, No. 5: 258-67.

HARRISON, J., C. JOHNSON, N. WEIZER et al. 1978. *A New Governance Structure for OCLC: Principles and Recommendations*. Metuchen (N.J.), London: Scarecrow Press.

OCLC Europe (and Membership). 1984. *VINE* No. 54: 17-21.

OCLC *Newsletter*. 1984-1996.

PLOTNIK, A. 1976. "OCLC for you and me? ! . . ." *American Libraries* 7, No. 5: 258-67.

OCLC. 1997. "What the OCLC Online Union Catalog means to me. A collection of essays." Dublin (OH).

OCLC in Latin America
and the Caribbean

Rosaly Favero Krzyzanowski
Inês Maria de Morais Imperatriz

INTRODUCTION

Before considering the great impact in the 1990s of library networking in Latin America in general and Brazil in particular, it is worthwhile to review briefly the recent history and nature of library services in these regions. Generally, libraries have followed international technological trends while concentrating their services on meeting the local needs of their patrons. However, the cooperative initiatives that are the focal point of modern library services have generally been lacking. It was very difficult for libraries with limited budgets and resources to keep pace with the continuing proliferation of information. Libraries began to look at computer technology as a way to automate and enhance their library services as well as modernize them. International institutions, such as the Organization of American States (OAS) and United Nations Educational, Scientific and Cultural Organization (UNESCO), as well as other sponsoring agencies within various Latin American and the Caribbean countries (LAC), started supporting library networking activities in the region.

Rosaly Favero Krzyzanowski is Technical Director, University of São Paulo Integrated Library System, Technical Department, São Paulo, Brazil.

Inês Maria de Morais Imperatriz is Division of Information Treatment Director, University of São Paulo Integrated Library System, Technical Department, São Paulo, Brazil.

[Haworth co-indexing entry note]: "OCLC in Latin America and the Caribbean." Krzyzanowski, Rosaly Favero, and Inês Maria de Morais Imperatriz. Co-published simultaneously in *Journal of Library Administration* (The Haworth Press, Inc.) Vol. 25, No. 2/3, 1998, pp. 159-176; and: *OCLC 1967-1997: Thirty Years of Furthering Access to the World's Information* (ed: K. Wayne Smith) The Haworth Press, Inc., 1998, pp. 159-176. Single or multiple copies of this article are available for a fee from The Haworth Document Delivery Service [1-800-342-9678, 9:00 a.m. - 5:00 p.m. (EST). E-mail address: getinfo@haworthpressinc.com].

Local, national and regional consortia were established to develop tools for libraries to meet the demands of the Information Age. This paper will focus on academic and research library networking in LAC, where a high level of library service has been achieved.

THE INFORMATION CHALLENGES OF THE 80s AND 90s TO LAC COUNTRIES

There is little mention of library services in LAC in the professional literature prior to the 1980s. Thereafter, a new generation of librarians in the region began expressing their concerns for improvement of library services. Among them was Saucedo Lugo (1983), who states that "Latin America is a region of sharp contrasts, and there are also sharp contrasts in library service among university libraries. The social, economic, political and cultural factors in the community in which the university is located and the general conditions of the country and of the university itself have a decisive influence on the status and characteristics of the university's library." She concludes that "The university library in Latin America is at an important stage of its development. Great progress has been made, but much remains to be done. Proper planning, backed up by qualified human resources and an adequate budget, will ensure that all university libraries in the region reach the standard of quality required to support the teaching, research and extension activities entrusted to the universities." Macedo (1988), based on three relevant papers (Saracevic, Braga and Quijano Solis, 1979; Almada Ascencio, 1982; Basic Principles . . . , 1986) and on her own reflections, states that although the idea of library cooperation was much discussed locally in the 60s and 70s, it took some time for this idea to become a reality in several Latin American countries, including Brazil. A variety of factors contributed to the delay in improving library services in the region. While developed countries were automating their library services, poor telecommunications and computer import restrictions were significant barriers to progress in the region. In addition, Macedo (1988) recommends that "before developing resource sharing plans, LAC countries need to develop closer relationships and get to know each other better in addition to studying ways to develop bibliographic tools needed to provide access to information."

Some years later, Lau (1995) reviewed resource sharing in the research libraries of Latin America and noted that "few regions of the world have as many things in common as Latin America (LA) in terms of language, religion and history. These similarities have fostered similar outlooks and attitudes among libraries in the region. However, despite this fact, it is difficult to generalize about libraries on the whole continent." He also says that: "Research and academic libraries are the most developed information centers in Latin America. . . . However, library collaboration and cooperation are limited, due primarily to poor telecommunication links."

It is worthwhile to point out that there are some sectors and regions in LAC that still present significant challenges to information managers who wish to access and use modern information technologies. To identify the populations involved, Cubillo (1997) proposes a metaphor consisting of an "iceberg," where: (a) at the tip is a small group of people and organizations who are in the vanguard and who can completely explore the worldwide resources available on the information superhighway, (b) in the middle is a larger group, mainly in the larger cities who are adopting the new information technologies, but who have not yet realized the full potential of these new resources, and (c) on the lowest layer is the largest group, invisible and below the water line, which consists of the vast majority of the people, from children to the elderly, from middle class to poor, for whom the new information technologies could have the most spectacular results if used appropriately.

In order to build cooperation among national information systems and networks for Latin American and the Caribbean, UNESCO has played a relevant role through its *General Information Programme* (PGI) (Fernández-Aballí, 1996). Among the various issues, a newsletter entitled INFOLAC[1] assembles and disseminates information on this area among all member countries.

Moreover, one regional institution, ECLAC (Economic Commission for Latin America and the Caribbean),[2] through its division CLADES (Latinamerican Center of Economic and Social Documentation),[3] by means of its *Program of Information Management,* has been developing outstanding seminars on this area throughout LAC, keeping permanent interaction with more than 180 organizations in 17 LAC countries (Alba, Gazitúa and Cubillo, 1997).

This context shows that some efforts have been developed to date, and adequate planning and management will lead to greater enhancement in information availability in LAC, through the use of modern technologies for the establishment of information networking.

NETWORKING IN LATIN AMERICA AND THE CARIBBEAN

Although information professionals faced many difficulties in modernizing library services in LAC, they have worked intensively at both technical and political levels to achieve integration, to cope with financial and cultural obstacles, and to prepare staff to meet the challenges of the Information Age. "In relation to information networks, Latin America and the Caribbean, in the last two decades, have promoted a group of initiatives in many fields deriving from the need to share information about research that is being done in the region." Some of these information networks include: REDUC (in education), INFOPLAN and CARISPLAN (in planning), INFOLAC (in cooperation between networks and national information systems), BIREME (in health sciences), DOCPOL (in population research), CLAD (in public administration), CLACSO (in social sciences), REPIDISCA (in sanitary engineering) (Cabezas, 1995). Most of them use the software packages CDS/ISIS, distributed by UNESCO and prepared specially for developing countries. Furthermore, there have been many professional meetings in the region to discuss common problems and to achieve stronger interaction among network and information systems administrators (Hahn, 1995). Based on the scenario described in the previous section, some changes had to be made to the usual mechanisms of information management. However, according to Cubillo (1997), the changes inherent in the *Pre*-Internet world would not be the same in the *Post*-Internet world. The leadership[4] of information managers will be an essential factor in the transition. Gazitúa (1997), writing about the information management environment in LAC, notes that in recent years new conditions, such as the Internet, allowed the connection to information networks in different patterns. There have been changes in telecommunications and in market regulations and advances in computer science such as the development of open systems and personal computing. As a result, he points out that *the technological environment shows that **almost all limitations have been overcome, and the great responsibility to achieve progress lies more on the information agents than on the technologies.***

Internet access in LAC shows an exponential growth in the region (Table 1), providing a strong base to develop plans for modernizing of library services. Once international patterns and standards are also adopted, it will be possible to enhance cooperative actions among LAC and foreign countries via the Internet. Also, LAC libraries can benefit from international library services such as cataloging and reference that are available over the Internet.

Cabezas (1995), studying Internet potential for services in Latin America, states that "clearly, 1994 marks the year of consolidation or integration of numerous national networks in Latin America and the Caribbean into the global Internet." He also adds: "Today the word is interconnectiv-

TABLE 1. Growth of Internet Hosts in Latin America and the Caribbean*
(January 95/97)

Country	Jan 95	Jan 96	Jan 97
Brazil	800	20,113	77,148
Mexico	6,656	13,787	29,840
Chile	3,054	9,027	15,885
Argentina	1,262	5,312	12,688
Colombia	1,127	2,262	9,054
Peru	171	813	5,192
Costa Rica	798	1,495	3,491
Venezuela	529	1,165	2,417
Dom. Rep.	**	139	2,301
Uruguay	172	626	1,823
Panama	17	148	751
Ecuador	325	504	590
Nicaragua	49	141	531
Bolivia	**	66	430
Honduras	***	***	408
Guatemala	**	27	274
Jamaica	76	164	249
Bahamas	**	276	195 (sic)
Paraguay	**	85	195
Antigua	**	163	169
Trinidad & Tobago	55	66	141
El Salvador	23	43	132
Dominica	**	27	55
Guyana	–	3	52
St. Lucia	–	20	21
Barbados	–	9	21
Suriname	–	2	4
St. Kitts	–	**	22

*   Source: OAS/RedHUCyT (Network Wizards (http://www.nw.cm)) – (Office of . . . , 1997)
**   Countries connected to the Internet after January of respective year.
*** Connected after May 1995.

ity via the Internet and there is a unique opportunity to take advantage of these infrastructures."

In addition, some aspects of network connectivity related to the local environment are included below.

Sadowsky (1993), considering the network connectivity for developing countries, points out that these countries as a whole are quite heterogeneous, and that "any general statement that one makes for developing countries as a class can almost always be contradicted by specific examples." He presents a division of those countries in "lesser developed countries" and "developing countries at a more advanced stage of development" for the purpose of digital network development. He also declares that: ". . . it is increasingly likely that the idea of developing countries helping themselves can be realized in a time-efficient manner. In order to maximize such a payoff, developing countries must be prepared to have their representatives immerse themselves in the culture of electronic networking and learn how to make it work for their national development."

Lynch (1994) also describes the exponential growth of Internet traffic in Latin America in the face of such obstacles as insufficient communication networks, legal impediments, and high costs of international connections. Despite these obstacles, academic networks are being created throughout Latin America and they are using the Internet for access to electronic mail, videoconferencing, supercomputers, databases and international programs and a wide range of interactive communications. Many of the existing connections use PAS-1 Satellite, from Pan American Satellite Corporation, in order to communicate with NSFNet in Homestead, in Florida (Figure 1).

Moreover, Lau (1995) states: "New information technologies and the integration of regional and national computer networks, together with their connection to the Internet, have a great potential for increasing communication and cooperation among libraries in LA, as well as improving ties with their North American counterparts."

Hahn (1995) studied networking in Latin America and the Caribbean and the support of OAS, focusing on the RedHUCyT ("Hemisphere-Wide Inter-University Scientific and Technological Information Network") Project,[5] which started in 1991. Its main objective is "to connect the member countries to the Internet, by integrating an electronic network for the exchange of specialized information among different academic and scientific institutions in the member States." In the *Plan of Action* signed by 34 heads of States in 1994, during the "Summit of the Americas" held in Miami, Florida, those governments "recognize that a country's information infrastructure is an essential component of political, economic, social and cultural development." The Governments assume several key responsibilities including to encourage major universities, libraries, hospitals and government agencies to have access to these networks, building on the work of the OAS RedHUCyT project. This network has presently reached several LAC regions, as shown in Table 2.

FIGURE 1

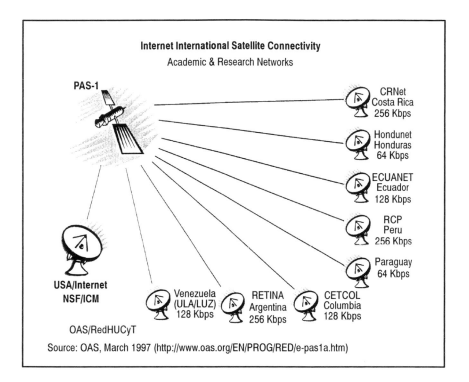

Source: OAS, March 1997 (http://www.oas.org/EN/PROG/RED/e-pas1a.htm)

Khouri (1996), presenting the major changes that have occurred in academic and research libraries at a seminar in Chile, states that "technology and telecommunications solved a series of problems, but they are generating new challenges that we have to deal with–'CCCP.' They stand for: Connectivity, Cooperation, Coordination and Partnership."

Carty (1997), studying the challenges of academic networks in Latin America (primarily in Colombia), identified three main barriers: (1) crisis in Latin America higher education; (2) publications and policy failure that pits PTTs (Post, Telegraph and Telephone, national communication utilities) against academic networks; and (3) centralization and the need to develop a culture of information. He offered a set of policy recommendations, including:

1. Academic networks must become embedded, conceptually and institutionally, in the current Latin American higher education reform process.

2. Academic networkers need to balance their well-justified preoccupation with uncooperative PTTs and national governments with a greater concern for the higher education reform movements.
3. University heads and the agencies that give them money need to make LAN (Local Area Network) development and IT training of personnel a priority.
4. Policy makers in Latin America need to develop integrated information infrastructure policies in order to stop pitting their PTTs against their academic and research networks.

TABLE 2. RedHUCyT* Member Countries and Academic & Research Networks (Updated March 1997)**

Region	Member Countries	Academic & Research Networks / Opening year
Andean Countries	Bolivia Colombia Ecuador Peru Venezuela	BOLNet (1995) CETCOL (1994) ECUANET RCP (1994) REACCIUN (1997)
Caribbean University Network (CUNet)	Jamaica * * *	JAMNet (1994)
MERCOSUL** countries and Chile**	Argentina Brazil Chile Paraguay Uruguay	RETINA RNP (1991) REUNA (1994) (1996) LATU
Mexico and Central America	Costa Rica *** El Salvador Guatemala Honduras Nicaragua Panama Mexico	CRNet (1996) SVNet (1996) MAYANet (1995) HONDUNet (1995) RAIN (1994) PANNet (1996) CONACYT

* Hemisphere Wide Inter-University Scientific and Technological Information Network

** Source: OAS (http://www.oas.org/EN/PROG/RED/covere.htm)

*** Projects for other countries in implementation stage

****MERCOSUL (South American Common Market, signed up in 1991 by Argentina, Brazil, Paraguay and Uruguay)

Besides the possibilities of maximizing access to worldwide information for LAC users, it is worth mentioning that use of the Internet is leading to another significant achievement for South American libraries–cooperation among regional, national and international union catalogs and networks in order to store their local bibliographic information based on common standards and patterns. Assuming that environmental difficulties will be overcome, it is possible to foresee that joint efforts towards common purposes in information management in LAC will produce similar results to those already obtained in developed countries (Commission of . . . , 1990), based on connectivity, cooperation, coordination and partnership.

BRAZILIAN INFORMATION SERVICES OVERVIEW

The picture of Latin American academic libraries, as presented by Saucedo Lugo (1983), can also be applied to Brazil: "Some major efforts have recently been made to centralize library activities and processes with a view to establishing information systems and networks. This trend is fostering interlibrary co-operation, is remedying some of the existing shortcomings and is facilitating the development and improvement of university libraries."

Frederick (1989), in a survey of university library programs' cooperative cataloging initiatives, identified problems associated with online network implementation in Brazil but offered a positive prognosis for Brazilian libraries to participate in other library networks.

Ferreira (1994) reviews the history of IBICT[6] and recommends strategies and goals for libraries for dealing with the effects of technology on Brazilian society. He notes that countries with an established information infrastructure started from three basic points: (1) good research and academic libraries, as well as excellence centers in specific areas; (2) databases and information networks and data communication; and (3) provision of information services. He argues that information services are the great strategic link–the true interconnecting channel between the academic source that produces knowledge and the potential users in the private sector.

In 1989, it was possible for Brazilian institutions to begin connecting to the Internet. Vargas (1994), in an analysis of local information and electronic networks, stated that implementation of the RNP (Rede Nacional de Pesquisa, the Brazilian Research Network, created in 1989, is the Brazilian branch of Internet) provided the scientific and technological community not only with faster access to worldwide information, but also accelerated scholarly communication and integration with their peers in Brazil and abroad. Since then, the RNP has spread throughout Brazil, and interest in international trade and commerce has made it a networking leader in the western hemisphere (Table 2 and Figure 2).

In the *Information Society in Brazil* (1997), Lucena and Campos discuss the role of the National Science and Technology Council (CNPq). They identify three conditions that must exist for a country to participate actively in the Information Age: (a) development of a national information infrastructure; (b) connection of that infrastructure to the worldwide information networks; and (c) improvement of human resources, a mandatory condition for the maintenance of a knowledge-based society.

THE UNIVERSITY OF SÃO PAULO
INTEGRATED LIBRARY SYSTEM (USP/SIBi)

One Brazilian institution that has recently connected to the international library networking community is the University of São Paulo (USP).

FIGURE 2

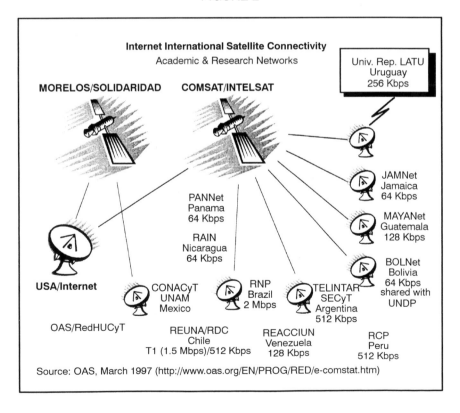

Founded in 1934 by the State of São Paulo, USP has 4,970 faculty, 55,250 students and 14,790 administrative staff on its six campuses which contain teaching and research units, specialized centers and institutes, hospitals, museums, and central management. It has an Integrated Library System, USP/SIBi (http://www.usp.br/sibi/sibi.html), composed of 38 libraries, a Technical Department and a Supervisory Council; its mission is to provide library services for the university objectives of teaching, research and extension.

Since 1985 USP/SIBi has been involved in developing library automation and in 1993 connected DEDALUS, its bibliographic database, to the Internet.

In 1997, with funding provided by the Fundação de Amparo à Pesquisa do Estado de São Paulo (FAPESP) (Krzyzanowski, Imperatriz and Rosetto, 1996), there was a major updating and enhancement of the USP/SIBi system with new hardware and software. A new client/server architecture now provides integrated library functions for the 38 libraries in the system. The main purpose of the upgrade was to improve library services and information access to meet research and teaching needs at the University of São Paulo and prepare the university to connect, cooperate and partner with similar institutions and organizations.

Other initiatives, such as agreements and cooperative activities at national and international levels, have also contributed to the enhancement of library services. USP/SIBi has participated in IBICT programs such as Catálogo Coletivo Nacional de Publicações Seriadas (CCN); Rede ANTARES, which promotes the sharing of science and technology databases at Brazilian institutions; Sistema de Informação sobre Teses (SITE) and Programa de Comutação Bibliográfica (COMUT). USP/SIBi also participates in regional union catalogs such as Catálogo Coletivo de Livros do Estado de São Paulo and UNIBIBLI-CD-ROM, a joint effort of the three State universities of the State of São Paulo. USP/SIBi is involved in LAC regional databases devoted to specific fields, such as LILACS/BIREME, in health sciences, and in conservation/preservation programs of the National Library. USP/SIBi participates in the international union catalog of OCLC WorldCat (the OCLC Online Union Catalog) as well as in regional IberoAmerican Science and Technology Education Consortium (ISTEC) for the use of LIGDOC for the exchange of full text of documents through the Internet.

OCLC AND USP/SIBI

During the planning of automation renewal at USP/SIBi, some international library tools and services were investigated at the national and international levels (Barry, Griffiths and Lundeen, 1995), and it was possible to obtain the most suitable solutions for USP information system demands that would complement the hardware and software acquisitions. One of those solutions was OCLC computer services. OCLC is a nonprofit computer library service and research organization that is "dedicated to public purposes of furthering access to the world's information and reducing information costs" (OCLC Online Computer Library Center, 1995/96). USP/SIBi was the first Brazilian institution to be visited by the newly established OCLC Latin America and the Caribbean Division in 1995.

Initially, USP/SIBi is enhancing the technical services area to strengthen the base for its other library services. DEDALUS records, which contained a limited number of fields, were expanded to the full MARC format in the new system. Simultaneously, with funding from the A. W. Mellon Foundation, USP contracted with OCLC for a 600,000-title retrospective conversion project for monograph records from the DEDALUS database. Fifty-five percent of the records were converted using OCLC's DDR/FullMARC (Duplicate Detection and Resolution/FullMARC) software and then migrated into the DEDALUS database, implemented by ALEPH software (produced by EX-LIBRIS, an Israeli-based company). In addition, USP/SIBi agreed to do all its current cataloging on the OCLC system, thereby becoming the first OCLC member library in Brazil to participate in OCLC online shared cataloging. In that same spirit of cooperation, USP/SIBi has made preliminary arrangements with the Library of Congress to participate in the *NACO* (National Coordinated Cataloging Operations) program.

OCLC services are enabling USP/Sbi to:

- Build and to enrich local machine-readable catalogs in full MARC format much more rapidly and consistently
- Reduce the staff labor of cataloging
- Save cataloging costs
- Guarantee quality of records by using an international bibliographic database, WorldCat, that is kept under a permanent quality control program
- Contribute original cataloging of local bibliographic information to WorldCat
- Be a member of the world's largest and most comprehensive database of bibliographic information
- Obtain technical support for USP librarians training, as well as for the development of USP/SIBi planned activities in cooperation and retrospective conversion.

As a consequence, the USP/SIBi database will be technically updated and enriched in its contents, and librarians will be much more skilled in technical tasks, as well as in reference searching and access to information to meet users' needs.

OCLC IN LATIN AMERICA AND THE CARIBBEAN

Now that Latin America and the Caribbean countries have succeeded in improving their telecommunications resources, it is time for information systems and network managers to plan the future of their institutions, based on international standards and patterns, in order to achieve world-wide connectivity. As it is quite impossible for any library to meet the information needs of its users with only its own resources, it is necessary to enhance the arrangements for cooperation and partnership with libraries in the region as well as to take advantage of international library computer services, such as those provided by OCLC.

The building of regional and national bibliographic databases under accurate bibliographic control will produce a variety of tools to fulfill users' needs and generally increase the availability of information in Latin America and the Caribbean. According to the 1996/97 OCLC Annual Report, WorldCat contains 1,525,107 records in Spanish and 304,811 in Portuguese. Certainly these numbers will increase as a result of more effective bibliographic control in the region and the production of records according to international standards. Also, access to information through the Internet will provide LAC users with information available worldwide, contributing to the development of research and teaching at educational institutions and other sectors of the information society.

Libraries in LAC can now use the Internet or CompuServe Global Data Communications to connect to the OCLC network. As new RedHUCyT academic and research information networks are established (Table 3), it is likely that they will increase their use of OCLC services in the future.

FINAL REMARKS

The enhancement of telecommunication resources in LAC countries will provide many benefits to information networks in the region. However, due to environmental differences, network managers will have to choose the solutions most appropriate to their region to achieve their goals. In making these choices, network planners would do well to keep these factors in mind:

TABLE 3. OCLC Products and Services at Latin American and Caribbean Institutions (Updated May 1997)

Region / Country	Institution	OCLC Products / Services*
ANDEAN COUNTRIES		
Colombia	Universidad de los Andes	FS
	Universidad Nacional de Colombia	CatCD
Venezuela	Banco Central de Venezuela	CatCD
CARIBBEAN COUNTRIES		
Barbados	University of the West Indies	CatOL, FS
Bermuda	Bermuda Biological Station for Research, Inc.	FS
Jamaica	University of the West Indies	CatOL, CatCD, FS
	University of the West Indies, Department of Library and Information Sciences	CatCD, FS
Trinidad and Tobago	University of the West Indies	CatOL, CatCD, FS
MERCOSUL** COUNTRIES AND CHILE		
Brazil	Fundação Getulio Vargas	CatCD, FS
	Pontifícia Universidade Católica do Rio de Janeiro	CatCD, FS
	Universidade do Estado de Santa Catarina	FS
	Universidade Federal de Juiz de Fora	CatCD, FS
	Universidade Federal de Minas Gerais	
	– Biblioteca Central	CatCD, FS
	– Escola de Biblioteconomia	FS
	– Faculdade de Educação	FS
	Universidade Federal de Pernambuco	CatCD
	Universidade Est. Paulista "Julio de Mesquita Filho"	CatCD
	Universidade Estadual de Campinas	CatCD
	Universidade de São Paulo–Sistema Integrado de Bibliotecas	CatOL, Conversion
	Universidade Regional de Blumenau	FS
Chile	Pontifícia Universidad Católica de Chile	FS
	Universidade de Chile	
	– Dpto. Física	FS
	– Dpto. Quimica	FS
Uruguay	Universidad ORT (Organización de Recursos Educacionales y Entrenamiento Tecnológico)	FS

TABLE 3 (continued)

Region / Country	Institution	OCLC Products / Services*
MEXICO AND CENTRAL AMERICA		
Costa Rica	Banco Central de Costa Rica	FS
	Instituto Costarricense de Electricidad–Centro Informacion Energética	FS
	Instituto Centroamericano de Administración de Empresas	FS
	Universidad Nacional	CatCD, FS
El Salvador	Biblioteca Manuel Gallardo	CatCD
Mexico	Benemerita Universidad Autonoma de Puebla	CatOL, FS
	CETYS Universidad, Campus Mexicali	CatCD, FS
	CETYS Universidad, Campus Tijuana	FS
	Escuela de Graduados en Liderazgo Empresarial	FS
	Universidad de las Americas	FS
	Universidad Autonoma de Ciudad Juarez	FS
	Universidad Autonoma Metropolitana– Azcapotzalco	SS, FS
	Universidad Nacional Autonoma de Mexico	FS
	Universidad de Sonora	
Nicaragua	Instituto Centroamericano de Administracion de Empresas	FS

* Source of OCLC Products/Services in LAC = OCLC Latin American and the Caribbean Division (Personal communication). OCLC Products/Services codes:

CatCO   =   CatCD for Windows cataloging using CO-ROM

CatOL   =   Cataloging Oniine

FS   =   FirstSearch

SS   =   SiteSearch

Conversion =   Retrospective Conversion/DDR FullMARC

* * MERCOSUL (South American Common Market, signed up in 1991 by Argentina, Brazil, Paraguay and Uruguay)

Considering the same regional distribution of RedHUCyT member countries (Table 1), this table shows that OCLC has products and services in all LAC regions and in the majority of countries, enabling them to improve their services, either locally using CD-ROM, or online through Intemet connections.

- Increased demand for information in the region
- Need for bibliographic control of LAC publications
- Inclusion of LAC materials in national and international information databases
- Interconnection of regional and national databases
- Planning the future of libraries–collection management and preservation, maximization of information access, enhancement of information networks, and cooperative work
- Improvement of resource sharing and exchange of data among institutions
- Use of reliable library computer services to strengthen library tools and services
- Training of library professionals to deal with technology-based information, and also of end users to carry out their work
- Increased responsibility of information agents to achieve progress
- Creation of innovative programs of information marketing
- Evaluation of use of network systems in order to redesign them for end-users

NOTES

1. *INFOLAC*, a quarterly newsletter of the Regional Programme for Strengthening Co-operation among National Information Systems and Networks for Latin America and the Caribbean, is published under the auspices of the Information and Informatics Division (INF/LAC) of UNESCO/Caracas and the National Library of Venezuela.

2. *ECLAC* corresponds to *CEPAL* (*Comisión Económica para América Latina y el Caribe*).

3. *CLADES* (*Centro Latinoamericano de Documentación Económica y Social*) is a division of *CEPAL*.

4. *ECLAC* has been devoted to enhancing the understanding of the phenomena related to information management and leadership in LAC information systems, and is opened to joint efforts with other regional and international organizations in this search, whose results may determine the future development of LAC.

5. *RedHUCyT* (*Red Hemisferica Inter-Universitaria de Información Cientfica y Tecnológica*)

6. *IBICT* (*Instituto Brasileiro de Informação em Ciência e Tecnologia*)–Brazilian Institute of Information in Science and Technology, which was created in 1954, now settled in Brasilia, is responsible for the national information policies and relevant information programs in the country.

REFERENCES

Alba, Luis, José Miguel Gazitúa, and Julio Cubillo. 1997. *Tres enfoques sobre el nuevo gestor de la información.* Santiago de Chile, CEPAL/CLADES: 63 pp. (Información y Desarrollo, 8).

Almada Ascencio, Margarita. 1982. "Tecnologia de hoje: o ponto de vista do Terceiro Mundo." *Revista Latinoamericana de Documentación* 2 (2): 20-3.

Barry, Jeff, José-Marie Griffiths, and Gerald Lundeen. 1995. "The changing face of automation." *Library Journal* 120 (6): 44-54.

Basic principles for a regional programme to strengthen co-operation among national information networks and systems for development in Latin America and the Caribbean (Infolac). 1986. Santiago, Chile, UNESCO/PGI and CEPAL/CLADES: 79 pp.

Cabezas, Alberto. 1995 "Internet: potential for services in Latin America." *Infolac* 8 (2): 39-42.

Carty, Winthrop. 1997. "Challenges to academic networks in Latin America: the case of Colombia's Red CETCOL." Available at: http://som.csudh.edu/fac/lpress/devnat/nations/colombia/challenge/

Commission of the European Communities. 1990. "Plan of action for libraries in the EC. Action line 1." *IFLA Journal* 16 (1): 64-66.

Cubillo, Julio. 1997. "La búsqueda de nuevos liderazgos organizacionales en gestión de la información en América Latina y El Caribe." In: Alba, Luis, José Miguel Gazitúa, and Julio Cubillo. 1997. *Tres enfoques sobre el nuevo gestor de la información.* Santiago de Chile, CEPAL/CLADES: 47-61.

Fernández-Aballí, Isidro. 1996. "La información: un recurso esencial para el desarrollo." *Infolac* 9 (3): 3-10.

Ferreira, José R. 1994. "O impacto da tecnologia da informação sobre o desenvolvimento nacional." *Ciência da Informação* 23 (1): 9-15.

Frederick, Janet. 1989. "The birth of a network: the Brazilian struggle." *College and Research Libraries* 50 (1): 76-82.

Gazitúa, José Miguel. 1997. "Gestores de información y el entorno: algunas referencias para la navegación." In: Alba, Luis, José Miguel Gazitúa, and Julio Cubillo. 1997. *Tres enfoques sobre el nuevo gestor de la información.* Santiago de Chile, CEPAL/CLADES: 29-44.

Hahn, Saul. 1997. "Networking in Latin America and the Caribbean and the OAS/RedHUCyT Project." Available at: http://www.isoc.org/HMP/PAPER/168/txt/paper.txt

Khouri, Anastassia. 1996. "Building a global information infrastructure: necessity to reengineer the academic library." In Conferencia Internacional de Bibliotecas de Educación Superior de América Latina y El Caribe, Santiago. *Ponencias.* Santiago, Colegio de Bibliotecarios de Chile.

Krzyzanowski, Rosaly F., Inês M.M. Imperatriz, and Marcia Rosetto. 1996. "Gestões para a modernização do Sistema Integrado de Bibliotecas da Universidade de São Paulo: incremento da automação através de projetos em desenvolvimento." In: Seminário Nacional de Bibliotecas Universitárias, 9., Curitiba. *Anais . . .* Curitiba, UFRP/PUCRP, Ref.6.6 (diskette)

Krzyzanowski, Rosaly F., Inês M.M. Imperatriz, and Marcia Rosetto. 1996 a. *Subsídios para análise, seleção e aquisição de software para gerenciamento de bibliotecas: experiência do Sistema Integrado de Bibliotecas da USP (SIBi/ USP)*. São Paulo, SIBi/USP: 56pp. (Cadernos de Estudos, 5)

Lau, Jesús. 1995. "Resource sharing in the research libraries of Latin America." In: *Annual Conference of Research Library Directors, 13, Dublin, Ohio. Proceedings*. Dublin, Ohio, OCLC: 21-26.

Lucena, Carlos J.P. and Ivan M. Campos. 1996. "A construção da *Sociedade da Informação* no Brasil: o papel do Conselho Nacional de Ciência e Tecnologia." In: Proposta de um Projeto para *A Sociedade da Informação no Brasil*. Versão Preliminar: 1-10.

Lynch, Karen. 1994. "Internet a la Latina." *Communications Week Latinoamerica/ Online/ Marzo 1994.*" Available at: http://ns.crnet.cr/documentos/karen.html

Macedo, Neusa D. 1988. "Cooperação na América Latina e Caribe para a área da informaçao documentária." *Revista brasileira de Biblioteconomia e Documentação*, 21(3/4): 130-74.

Office of Science and Technology. 1997. RedHUCyT. Available at: http://www. oas.org/EN/PROG/RED/covere.htm

OCLC Online Computer Library Center. 1995/96. *OCLC Annual Report 1995/96: Furthering access to the world's information*. Dublin, Ohio: OCLC: 52 pp.

Sadowsky, George. 1993. "Network connectivity for developing countries." *Communications of the ACM*: 43-47.

Saracevic, Tefko, Gilda Braga, and Alvaro Quijano Solis. 1979. "Information systems in Latin America." *Annual Review of Information Science and Technology*, 24: 249-82.

Saucedo Lugo, María Elena. 1983. "University libraries in Latin America." *UNESCO Journal of Information Science, Libraries and Archives Administration* 5(2): 100-3.

Vargas, José I. 1994. "A informação e as redes eletrônicas." *Ciência da Informação* 23 (1): 7-8.

The Transformation from Microfilm to Digital Storage and Access

Meg Bellinger

INTRODUCTION

Digital imagery is revolutionizing the traditional concepts of preservation and access in libraries and archives. Preservation has been clearly defined and understood for the last twenty years by a set of widely accepted treatments. And while these treatments have provided a strong level of assurance for the perpetuity of the original or the surrogate, the result often has been a limitation placed on access. Digital imaging promises more universal access, at the cost, however, of a decline in the level of security in the preservation of the original or a reasonable surrogate.

ANALOG PRESERVATION

Preservation of paper-based materials entails either the stabilization of the original artifact and the subsequent control of its environment (the creation of a surrogate to reduce use of the original and thereby perpetuate its existence), or, when the original is unstable, the transfer of the intellectual content to another, more stable medium to ensure availability of information in the new medium.

For the past two decades, high-volume preservation efforts and funding

Meg Bellinger is President, Preservation Resources, Bethlehem, PA.

[Haworth co-indexing entry note]: "The Transformation from Microfilm to Digital Storage and Access." Bellinger, Meg. Co-published simultaneously in *Journal of Library Administration* (The Haworth Press, Inc.) Vol. 25, No. 4, 1998, pp. 177-185; and: *OCLC 1967-1997: Thirty Years of Furthering Access to the World's Information* (ed: K. Wayne Smith) The Haworth Press, Inc., 1998, pp. 177-185. Single or multiple copies of this article are available for a fee from The Haworth Document Delivery Service [1-800-342-9678, 9:00 a.m. - 5:00 p.m. (EST). E-mail address: getinfo@haworthpressinc. com].

have been focused on reformatting or copying information from unstable originals to media with proven and verifiable standards for longevity. For paper-based materials, this has meant primarily preservation microfilming. Standards for quality reproduction of the content of the original and for ensuring the technical quality and longevity of the medium for preservation microfilm are clearly defined and testable, universally accepted and rigorous. Such standards for digital imaging for preservation quality have not been defined.

A significant investment of resources has been made in the preservation of library and archive materials in microform. Microformats have been the primary medium of choice for media conversion of large quantities of library materials. By mid-1994, it is estimated that the NEH Brittle Book program has preserved on microfilm 654,000 volumes or 98.1 million frames. The U.S. Newspaper Program has funded the filming of 220,000 titles and 53 million frames. The goal is for the program to film 2 million volumes, or 300 million frames in 20 years (by the year 2009).

Much of this work has been done by Preservation Resources, originally called MAPS, the Mid-Atlantic Preservation Service. The organization was founded in 1985 to serve preservation microfilming needs by five mid-Atlantic research libraries–Columbia University Libraries, Cornell University Library, Princeton University Library, New York State Library, and the New York Public Library.

A division of OCLC since January 1994, Preservation Resources now operates from a custom-designed laboratory in Bethlehem, Pennsylvania built with funds from the Pew Charitable Trust. Preservation Resources serves the preservation needs of clients from every part of North America and increasingly is reaching a global client base. The infrastructure and operating principles were formulated and implemented by information professionals, and the organization continues to be operated by librarians seeking continual improvements and preservation options to meet the needs of information professionals engaged in the effort to preserve and provide access to our cultural heritage.

Microfilm's stable and standardized properties and its convertibility to other media will guarantee its continued use in the preservation community for reformatting for decades to come. However, microfilm ultimately is viewed as a medium of storage rather than of access. With the increased availability of computer workstations in the library and with researchers remotely connected through the Internet, electronic access to research materials is a concept whose time has arrived.

DIGITAL PRESERVATION

The library and archive community is currently engaged in defining standards or best practices for converting research materials to digital format. Questions of quality, authenticity, validation and metadata requirements are being addressed. The question of the preservation of the medium will only be addressed through a universally accepted means of archival storage, with assurance of periodic migration of digital information.

In addition to questions of quality to ensure that the intellectual content of the original is represented in the digital image, questions remain about preserving the systems in which images are stored, viewed, and transmitted.

The current pace of technological change is staggering. Backward compatibility from software and media generations are only promised by some technology providers. Media selected for the transfer and preservation of information must, by definition, provide greater stability and longevity than the original medium.

Preservation microfilming produces one master and subsequent generations for copying or for use. Each generation represents some loss of fidelity. However, if properly produced and stored, silver halide microfilm has a life expectancy of 500 years.

Digital images may be copied repeatedly without loss of fidelity as long as the media upon which it is stored remains stable and the equipment and software required to open and copy the image is available. Estimates published in the "Storage Technology Assessment Report," by the National Media Lab in 1994 put the life expectancy of optical media (CD-ROM, magneto Optico, and WORM) at anywhere from five to 100 years, depending upon manufacture and storage conditions. Magnetic tape is given a life expectancy of two to 30 years.

Given the extreme variability of these estimates, as Jeff Rothenburg stated in his article, *Ensuring the Longevity of Digital Documents,* "It is only slightly facetious to say that digital information lasts forever–or five years, whichever comes first."

Rothenburg's concern goes well beyond the question of the longevity of media to the very hardware, processes, and software used to write the digital information to the media and to store and retrieve the digital information. Estimates vary, but rates of hardware and software obsolescence can be anywhere from two to five years.

Data refreshment and migration have been posed as the only reliable methods to address the problems of technological obsolescence. Refreshment is the act of copying from one medium to another; however, given the life expectancy of optical and magnetic media cited above, and the astonishing rate of technological obsolescence, migration–the movement of information content from obsolete systems to current hardware and software systems so that information remains accessible and usable–is considered the more robust method to ensure the preservation of digital information.

In the Task Force report, migration is defined "as a set of organized tasks designed to achieve the periodic transfer of digital materials from one hardware/software configuration to another, or from one generation of computer technology to a subsequent generation. The purpose of the migration is to retain the ability to display, retrieve, manipulate and use digital information in the face of constantly changing technology. Migration includes refreshing as a means of digital preservation but differs from it in the sense that it is not always possible to make an exact digital copy or replica of a database or other information object, inasmuch as hardware and software change and still maintain the compatibility of the object with a new generation of technology" (p. 4).

Digitization is a reality which already provides a wider and immediate access to research materials than is possible in analog formats, but digital imaging is not yet preserving until the infrastructure is in place to assert that digital products meet the stated goal–whether of access or preservation, but ideally of both.

The traditional definitions of preservation no longer hold in the digital image context. A major function of preservation in the paper-based world has been to ensure longevity through managing the artifact. By necessity this has been a reactive effort. Whereas universities and libraries have been repositories of information, they are now largely the creators of image collections. This translates into greater opportunity, as well as greater responsibility for ensuring that preservation concerns are addressed as part of the process. The responsibility, fiscal commitment, and managerial control required to move terabytes of data on a two- to five-year cycle are daunting. Nevertheless, this is the most significant problem to be resolved if digital imaging is to be viewed as a preservation option.

OCLC AND PRESERVATION RESOURCES

Since early 1996, OCLC has been engaged in a research and demonstration project to prove the viability of a centralized electronic archive. OCLC's mission to serve the library community, its fiscal health and vast computing infrastructure, point to a leading role in the development of a centralized digital archive where assurances of periodic migration will guarantee the preservation of digital information. OCLC's activity in Electronic Archiving along with the development of best practices for digitization in the library and archive community, will allow Preservation Resources to develop services for direct digital imaging of research materials.

With a decade of experience in preservation project planning and implementation, micrographic technology, high-quality microfilm production, and the preservation of multiple documentary formats, Preservation Resources now is engaged in producing digital images of research materials. Digital imaging from preservation microfilm of research materials is an emerging technology. Preservation Resources is at the forefront of providing the expertise and services to make the intelligent translation from one medium to the next.

The Preservation Resources laboratory, a 17,150-square-foot facility built in 1990, was designed specifically to meet Preservation Resources' production and security requirements and is the most technically sophisticated micrographic operation in the country. The camera studio is equipped with 13 state-of-the-art, high resolution, computer-controlled Herrmann and Kraemer (H&K) cameras. Coupled with ExpoSure™, Preservation Resources' patented exposing system, the organization is producing film of unparalleled quality. The cameras operate on three shifts and have a production capacity of over 14 million frames per year. This is equivalent to 14,000 reels of microfilm or the potential to preserve 70,000 brittle volumes annually.

Since its inception, Preservation Resources has filmed well over 20 million frames of preservation quality microfilm. Preservation Resources' efforts to date translate into approximately 200,000 volumes microfilmed and preserved. Preservation Resources has served hundreds of institutions, including the preservation programs of large research libraries, academic library special collections, and also smaller institutions such as local historical societies, archives, and museums.

Preservation Resources has successfully filmed a variety of materials including embrittled monographs, pamphlets and serials, bound and unbound newspapers, manuscript collections, scrapbooks, technical drawings, and photographs. Among 20 other projects, we are currently filming large NEH-funded brittle book projects for the New York Public Library (History of the Americas project), SOLINET (ASERL project), Princeton University (Arabic Collection), University of Notre Dame (Medieval Institute) and Columbia University (Modern Economic and Social History). These comprehensive, large-scale, multi-year projects help Preservation Resources to refine procedures and schedules and to develop consistent experience which contributes to cost-savings.

At OCLC, efforts are underway to establish costs for archiving and making digital images available through online (or "near-line") access. This large-scale "electronic archiving pilot project" will demonstrate to libraries, publishers, and users the capabilities of storing large collections of digitized information and facilitating access in a very cost-effective manner.

In undertaking this project, collections utilizing a variety of original formats (e.g., newspapers, journals, photographs, etc.) have been selected, which were also chosen with the intention that these presentations will be of interest to a wide audience. As part of this important initiative, Preservation Resources has begun the scanning and indexing of three unique collections–involving an estimated 100,000 images (out of the project's anticipated total of 250,000 images).

Digitization offers several advantages for the distribution of information. Scanned images can be accessed from remote sites and they can be organized in a variety of ways as well as linked to other electronic media. Preservation Resources creates custom indices for scanned images that can be designed to provide immediate access, while offering page-level browsing and hot links to subject indices or finding aids.

Using two SunRise SRI-50 scanners, Preservation Resources scans microfilm images that can be saved in various file formats for use on the Internet, compact disc or tape storage. All standard film formats can be converted to high-quality bitonal or grayscale digital images. Trained scanning technicians set up the ScanFlo™ scanner control software to best capture the images preserved on film. Adjustments are made for edge detection, thresholding, skew correction, and de-speckling, which are all particularly important for non-uniform projects, damaged materials or photograph-rich microfilm. Once images are scanned to a high capacity server, a network of five other Pentium workstations are used for quality assurance, post image processing and indexing.

These efforts are synergistic with OCLC's goal to develop a viable electronic archiving service to provide the library community with reliable storage and distribution options as collections are digitized. Several of Preservation Resources' scanning projects contribute directly to OCLC's electronic archive initiative, through which 12 institutions are collaborating with OCLC in a pilot project that tests electronic archiving technology. These projects include:

- *New York Public Library: Digital Schomburg.* The Schomburg Collection at the New York Public Library represents one of the premier collections of African Americana in the country. Nearly 22,000 pages from 65 titles have been scanned from microfilm. These include titles such as *Slave Life in Virginia and Kentucky,* written in 1863 by an escaped slave; travel narratives of the Americas and Africa; and a volume written in 1907 by Booker T. Washington. Images from this collection will be available in 1997.

- *Irish American Advocate.* Actor Carroll O'Connor has underwritten the preservation of an Irish American newspaper, *The Advocate,* which his grandfather, John C. O'Connor, founded in the late 19th century. Preservation Resources preserved the volumes on microfilm of all known issues from 1893 to 1988. The scanning of these 700+ issues resulted in 6.6 gigabytes of data. Headlines from these issues have been entered into a searchable database.
- *Civil War Regimental Histories. Knox College and Museum of the Confederacy.* Preservation Resources has scanned 24 volumes of regimental histories and books of Civil War campaigns, including reminiscences of volunteer regiments from Tennessee, Alabama, Iowa, Minnesota and Ohio; prisoner of war accounts; recollections of an army nurse; and histories of regiments composed of Black Americans.

Additional Preservation Resources projects that are part of OCLC's electronic archiving efforts include:

- Approximately 1,000 photographs from the Grand Rapids (Mich.) Public Library's Robinson Collection of "All American Girls Professional Baseball League."
- A journal on technology and railroads dating to the 19th century from the University of Illinois at Chicago, *Locomotive Engineering, a Practical Journal of Railway Motive Power and Rolling.* The scanning project included 41 volumes that were published from 1888 to 1928.
- A 20-volume set from Northwestern University, *The Writings and Speeches of the Right Honourable Edmund Burke.*

Preservation Resources Imaging Projects

Preservation Resources has been conducting research and development into digital imaging since 1991 with numerous research and demonstration projects. The culmination is the development of a scanning studio that parallels the organization's preservation microfilming activity. Preservation Resources has scanned many different formats from microfilm including monographs, serials, manuscripts, photographs and newspapers.

Currently, all digital projects undertaken by Preservation Resources originate from microfilm. So, while materials are made available electronically through scanning, they are also preserved on microfilm, which, properly processed and stored, has a projected life expectancy of 500 years.

Digital imaging projects include:

• *Library of Congress: NDL*

In August 1996, PresRes signed a contract with the Library of Congress to produce digital images of selected printed and manuscript collections from the Library's holdings. Approximately one million grayscale and bitonal images will be produced and made available by the National Digital Library Program over the Internet. The microfilm being scanned was produced between 1950 and 1994 and contains a diversity of challenges, including acetate and sprocketed originals, highly variable manuscript collections of 18th and 19th century origin. After much discussion on issues of quality and evaluation, the project began production in January and has produced 10,000 grayscale and 35,000 bitonal images to date. Images are delivered weekly on CD-ROM in JPEG and TIFF group IV file formats.

• *Columbia University Library: Museum Bulletin*

In 1996, Preservation Resources completed the scanning, image integration and indexing of Columbia University Libraries' *Museum Bulletin* project. Scanning was performed at 600 dpi and HTML Indexing links the image level to the table of contents. Samples of the images are available for viewing in Preservation Resources homepage (www.oclc.org/oclc/presres).

• *Association of Research Libraries: Presidential Messages*

In August 1995, Preservation Resources signed a contract with the Association of Research Libraries (ARL) to digitize from microfilm, index and write HTML for approximately 50,000 images on preservation microfilm of Mexican and Argentine Presidential Messages. The project will be complete in April 1997 with approximately 50 35mm reels scanned and 50,000 bitonal TIFF images indexed to three levels. The materials to be scanned are approximately 30 reels of Mexican and Argentine Presidential Messages. The content of the microfilm is 83 volumes of Mexican and 65 volumes of Argentine printed material originally published in the nineteenth and twentieth centuries. Page sizes range from $6''$ x $9''$ to $8''$ x $10''$

with approximately 90 percent in the 6″ x 9″ document size range. The material is primarily textual, with some charts and tables and a small number of illustrations. The images are available on the Internet through UT.

CONCLUSION

Libraries, archives, scholarly organizations, and publishers have already produced thousands, if not millions of digital images to increase access to research collections. These collections–from rare books from the Vatican to the letters of Emma Goldman–are allowing a heretofore unimagined level of access to a broad audience of connected users. The research and development efforts of OCLC and its preservation division will help to ensure that these collections will remain accessible for centuries to come.

The OCLC Institute:
Genesis and Prospectus

Martin Dillon

In 1997 the OCLC Board of Trustees established the OCLC Institute as a nonprofit educational organization dedicated to promoting the evolution of libraries and information services by providing managers with opportunities for advanced education and knowledge exchange. This article describes the genesis of the Institute, its mission and methods of operation and recent and near-term activities.

DEFINING THE NEED

Libraries and other information services are undergoing unprecedented changes, many of which are directly related to recent advances in computing and telecommunications technologies and their rapid and widespread adoption. The impact of technology is increasingly profound, changing the way we create, store, describe, distribute and access information, and the pace of change is accelerating. Traditional information media and organizational methods are giving way to emerging alternatives. Never before have libraries faced such multifaceted challenges nor been as pressured to provide new or increased services in a rapidly changing environment.

In addressing these challenges, library practices and management seem permanently in flux. Not surprisingly, this environment has placed signifi-

Martin Dillon is affiliated with OCLC Online Computer Library Center, Dublin, OH.

[Haworth co-indexing entry note]: "The OCLC Institute: Genesis and Prospectus." Dillon, Martin. Co-published simultaneously in *Journal of Library Administration* (The Haworth Press, Inc.) Vol. 25, No. 4, 1998, pp. 187-199; and: *OCLC 1967-1997: Thirty Years of Furthering Access to the World's Information* (ed: K. Wayne Smith) The Haworth Press, Inc., 1998, pp. 187-199. Single or multiple copies of this article are available for a fee from The Haworth Document Delivery Service [1-800-342-9678, 9:00 a.m. - 5:00 p.m. (EST). E-mail address: getinfo@haworthpressinc.com].

187

cant pressure on library education and the training of library professionals. L. Hunter Kevil, in an excellent article that exhorts library schools to become more adaptive, has expressed the challenge most succinctly, "For if the basic competencies required for library practice are in a flux, and what we have been taught is becoming obsolete, the very existence of the traditional library school will be highly problematic."[1] Kevil offers a new approach for the education of library professionals that, in effect, substitutes a complex of continuing education models for the traditional academic one.

Marilyn Miller, former dean at the University of North Carolina, Greensborough, makes a similar point:

> [W]e are constantly being confronted by graduates who tell us of the vastly more complicated work environment in which they operate. They must organize huge quantities of information resources within and outside the library. They must adapt quickly to new technologies. For instance, innovations involving computers–laptops, local-area and national networks, integrated systems, sophisticated online retrieval, CD-ROM databases, and interactive audiovisual systems such as computer-linked videodiscs–continue to transform the curriculum related to library information search, acquisition, retrieval, processing, and storage to an extent unimaginable a quarter century ago. And this is happening in all types of libraries, from the elementary school to the university.[2]

What is most interesting about the above is how little any of it reflects what has been the traditional content of library science education–cataloging formats and standards, classification theory, subject analysis, collection development and the like.

Library schools are not standing still, of course. As Miller points out, many have made energetic efforts to change.

> Upon reviewing the names of all forty-seven ALA-accredited programs, you will find that information science or information management dominates the choice of titles. So we now have an interesting collection of names. The University of California at Berkeley went through an historic upheaval three years ago and managed to survive, but their program name does not include the name "library" at all. Drexel has changed its name for the third time since the early eighties, when the "School of Library and Information Science" was superseded by "College of Information Studies." Effective July

1995, the name of the program is "College of Information Science and Technology."[3]

To Berkeley and Drexel can be added the School of Information at Michigan and the School of Information Studies at Syracuse, both innovative hybrids with an eye to the future.

While these changes are certainly healthy for the profession in the long term, it is not clear that they can immediately remedy the need for continuing education in the sense intended by Kevil. Additionally, it is not clear which of the many emerging models is the right one, or even if the concept of "right" is applicable. Schools of library and information science are changing their curricula, but the impact of new graduates in the workforce is insufficient for the current challenge: their numbers are too few, their skills are too unpracticed, and their ability to influence organizational change is too limited. All of these limitations, of course, are usually remedied by time, but time is of the essence. Drastically shortened technological life cycles do not allow libraries the luxury of time for a natural, generational renewal of professional skills as might be provided by traditionally matriculating students. New, dramatic and innovative approaches to ongoing professional training and education are needed.

Additional Evidence of Demand

Beginning in 1996, OCLC went through a strategic planning process that involved OCLC staff, the OCLC Users Council, OCLC's regionally affiliated Networks, the OCLC Board of Trustees and many OCLC advisory groups. An idea that repeatedly surfaced during this process was that OCLC contribute to solving the problem that libraries have in keeping abreast of technology. The U.S. Regional Networks particularly, all of which provide training for OCLC member libraries and others, were especially intense in stating that OCLC had a role to play in this area.

Coincidentally, representatives of BiblioData, a Brazilian network of libraries and a subsidiary of the Fundação Getulio Vargas (FGV), approached OCLC seeking help with an educational initiative for Brazilian librarians. The initiative was being funded by the Mellon Foundation and was aimed at providing a technology update for practicing librarians in Brazil. There were to be two parts: the first, a series of week-long seminars repeated a number of times across Brazil for as many mid-level library managers as could be accommodated; the second, a similar week-long seminar to be presented in the U.S. by appropriate experts with invited participants from Brazil drawn from the directors of the largest academic libraries. BiblioData sought OCLC's help because OCLC had recently begun to make available its services in Brazil. Over the years OCLC had been approached often with similar requests, but OCLC lacked the appropriate organization to respond in anything more than a piecemeal fashion.

As a consequence of all of these factors, OCLC management proposed at the November 18, 1996 board meeting that OCLC investigate the concept of establishing a permanent Institute with a mission to contribute to the continuing education of library professionals. The author was given the responsibility of carrying out this task, and in February 1997, the OCLC Board of Trustees approved the foundation of the OCLC Institute.

DEFINING THE SOLUTION

Defining a need for advanced library management education is a necessary but not sufficient cause for OCLC to found an educational institute. To succeed, such an institute must have a mission that is congruent with OCLC's purposes, possess unique resources that would be responsive to the educational needs of libraries, and fit within OCLC's operating structure.

The seeds for the OCLC Institute were planted decades ago with the drafting and adoption of the *OCLC Articles of Incorporation,* which, because of its significance as a guiding document, is worth reproducing here. According to the *Articles,* OCLC was formed:

> [T]o establish, maintain, and operate a computerized library network and to promote the evolution of library use, of libraries themselves, and of librarianship, and to provide processes and products for the benefit of library users, including such objectives as increasing the availability of library resources to individual library patrons and reducing the rate of rise of per-unit library costs, all for the fundamental public purpose of furthering ease of access to and use of the ever-expanding body of worldwide scientific, literary, and educational knowledge and information.[4]

Such promotion of library evolution is long evident in much of what OCLC has done and is doing by way of systems, services, products, and programs. The OCLC Institute represents a formalization of the intent to promote library evolution in additional ways.

The mission of the OCLC Institute is derived from OCLC's initial guiding purpose:

> The OCLC Institute is established as a nonprofit educational organization to promote the evolution of libraries and information services by providing managers with opportunities for advanced education and knowledge exchange.

This mission statement expresses the key components of the OCLC Institute and emphasizes the purposeful intent to facilitate change within libraries. This intent is motivated by a perceived need for advanced educational opportunities and for a more formal way of focusing OCLC resources toward this goal.

UNIQUE OCLC RESOURCES

The idea of an OCLC Institute is a natural one for many reasons having to do with OCLC's history and mission, partnerships, current capabilities, and physical plant. Throughout its history, OCLC has consistently contributed to the evolution of library processes and the education of practicing librarians in a variety of ways. Whether by supporting or helping to establish national standards or cooperative programs, OCLC has played a significant role in important national issues relating to librarianship. Similarly, OCLC has taken its place next to national and international library organizations in support of their goals. And not to be forgotten are OCLC's many interactions with vendors in the marketplace of information systems and services. Finally, and perhaps most notably, OCLC staff have frequently participated in conferences as panelists and speakers, not just to relay information on OCLC's products and services, but to speak more broadly on topics and issues that are of general concern to the library profession.

More formally, in recent years, OCLC has carried out a series of seminars as preconference activities to ALA Annual or Midwinter Meetings. The first of these, "The Future is Now: The Changing Face of Technical Services," held in 1994, dealt with evolving status of technical services and opened the question of outsourcing that function to discussion. Most recently, at the 1997 ALA Annual Meeting in San Francisco, a preconference was held that dealt with filtering mechanisms for accessing Internet resources. While these seminars have occasionally touched on OCLC services, their primary purpose has been to provide a forum for discussion of outstanding problems facing libraries that would benefit from open discussions.

OCLC's contribution to national dialogue is complemented by its corporate culture and accumulated base of knowledge. These are intangible but very real assets that depend on the superb OCLC staff. For the purposes of the OCLC Institute, two especially strong features of the staff are outstanding. The first is their service orientation, due equally to the role OCLC plays in helping libraries achieve their objectives–a blend of services and products that depend on a responsive staff at OCLC–and to the culture of librarianship which is shared strongly by OCLC staff, many of whom received their early professional training in libraries.

This point is underlined by a recent survey taken of the OCLC membership and is worth noting both in this context and for its own sake. The purpose of the survey was to register a baseline of membership satisfaction (or dissatisfaction) with OCLC's products and services. One feature of the survey results was a standout: the strong appreciation of respondents for the responsiveness of the OCLC staff. It is this same responsiveness that will make a strong contribution to the Institute's offerings because it encourages participation by the staff in helping members keep up-to-date on current technology.

But responsiveness, however attractive and useful, is not very helpful without a knowledge base to draw on. And here also, the OCLC staff is outstanding, both through their educational and technical background and also through their job responsibilities. OCLC, by necessity, is often required to be on the cutting edge of emerging technology, if not in its production facilities, then in its planning activities and research. Because the design and development cycles of new products remain long, staff must be intimately aware of next-generation technology long before it is actually in use to incorporate it into new products.

Two prime examples are available to us in recent OCLC product announcements. The first, OCLC FirstSearch Electronic Collections Online, made available in Spring 1997, captures the key critical concepts in the rapidly evolving field of electronic journal publication. This general field is crucial to the long-term planning and strategic evolution of libraries. How electronic journals are published and distributed will have a dramatic impact on library budgets, workflows and organizations. The OCLC solution, which will certainly continue to evolve in the next few years, arises from years of experimentation and research and is the culmination of its practical and theoretical experience. The knowledge and expertise that went into the design of the product are available to supplement the Institute's offerings. Indeed, it was included in the seminar presented to the Brazilian librarians referred to above.

A second example is the OCLC archiving experiment, which tests the concepts of centralized electronic archiving and near-line storage. It is clear that the library world is in for a long and perhaps agonizing search for an adequate means of preserving our cultural heritage in the age of electronic information. OCLC expects to be in the vanguard in this search and its archiving experiment is the first fruit of this quest. Again, the knowledge required to pursue this service is invaluable to course offerings through the Institute.

Many more examples could be cited: Internet cataloging, PURL technology, metadata research, PromptCat and outsourcing cataloging, SiteSearch technology and software–the list is lengthy. In each of these, OCLC has played a leadership role, one that can be strengthened and extended through the presentation of the underlying concepts and issues in Institute offerings.

To the extent that applied research, by expanding our knowledge of library problems and practices, participates in the educational process, OCLC's Office of Research has traditionally been the unit within OCLC that most contributes to the education of library professionals. Among its programs, four should be mentioned as particularly noteworthy in this respect. The first is its Visiting Scholar's program, where outstanding faculty are invited to spend a period of time at OCLC engaging in research of mutual interest. The second is the Library and Information Science Research Grant program, where OCLC annually awards research grants to projects undertaken by library school faculty. These are awarded through a competitive process and are designed more to advance the state of knowledge than to provide OCLC with answers to questions that advance its services. This year, for example, two grants were awarded where the research interest was information discovery on the Internet. The third is the Distinguished Seminar Series whereby noteworthy speakers are invited periodically to address a public gathering at OCLC to share current research or significant activities that impact librarianship. Apart from facilitating public discussion, these seminars help infuse the research environment at OCLC with new and creative ideas. Finally, OCLC's Office of Research publication program produces the *Annual Review of OCLC Research,* which has come to be relied upon as a primary method of disseminating the results of OCLC research and related activities.

The programs just described are in addition to the vital research program conducted by OCLC's research scientists, whose current investigations include metadata, automated subject analysis and classification, natural language processing and many aspects of digital libraries.

Finally, OCLC's physical plant provides the facilities necessary to support advanced education. Modern and comfortable meeting and training areas are equipped with computers and multimedia presentation systems. In addition, OCLC's production and research computing systems provide access to current and experimental software applications for use by instructors and students, and a full complement of desktop applications support the creation of educational products. Full-service training development, documentation, media resources, and printing/duplicating, which support OCLC's ongoing enterprise, are also available to support the OCLC Institute.

In summary, OCLC's long and active engagement with library issues, organizations, systems and services; its membership orientation and Network partnerships, its research and educational orientation, and its talented staff–by nature, training and job responsibility–and its substantial physical plant provide a unique reservoir of talent and capabilities to draw on in achieving its educational objectives.

DEFINING THE FUTURE

An awareness of the current technological climate informs the creation of the OCLC Institute and distills the following precepts:

- Libraries are undergoing fundamental, unprecedented change
- Opportunities for continued professional growth are essential for library and information services managers if they are to manage change successfully
- The challenge of meeting the needs of information professionals is very large and deserving of the best efforts of many organizations

The creation of the OCLC Institute, then, is OCLC's contribution to the broad and multifaceted field of advanced education and knowledge exchange for information managers.

Because the need for advanced educational opportunities is so great and the real resources that can be devoted to it are both limited and rare, the OCLC Institute will take great care not to duplicate what others are already doing well. Rather, the Institute will seek to exploit OCLC's own unique resources, to identify collaborative opportunities, and to develop partnerships that maximize the impact of combined resources.

As an initial step in defining its programs, the OCLC Institute surveyed a broad sample of libraries to solicit their views regarding its mission and programs.

A number of program types were investigated, primarily to understand what formats were attractive to potential attendees. The key variables were length of event, ranging from one day to one week, location, and cost. Not surprisingly, there was a clear preference for events held in regional locations, where an attendee did not have to travel far. This preference reinforces an existing inclination for the Institute to work closely with U.S. Regional Networks, complementing and expanding their offerings. A second preference, with respect to location, were events held in close proximity to national conferences such as ALA's annual conference. Since potential attendees were already traveling, the incremental cost of arriving early to attend a preconference event was minimal. While there is always a natural preference for events that are brief, with many favoring a day to a day and a half as a limit, substantial interest was expressed in seminars that were more lengthy. This is noteworthy because it allows for much more depth of presentation, a realistic need for many topics that might be offered by the institute.

A constant theme reiterated by many of the respondents was the primary importance of the topic. If the topic was of high interest, price and location were secondary, though in comparisons these factors predominated. When asked to recommend topics, respondents mentioned virtually all topics dealing with the Internet or electronic publication. Other frequently suggested topics include strategic planning, cost analysis and collection management.

International Needs. Because of the pressures of time and geography, our discussions with librarians about their precise needs and desires for increased educational opportunities were restricted primarily to the continental United States. Our knowledge of the educational needs of librarians beyond our borders needs additional intelligence. Nevertheless, it is clear that for developing countries, at least, the need for supplemental educational opportunities is very great. Equally great are the growing opportunities for developing countries to jump generations in terms of computing and telecommunications capabilities. Concomitant leaps in library and information management, however, are not nearly so obvious due in many cases to the lack of library traditions, cultural orientation toward information or government policy. In this regard, therefore, the sharing of U.S. expertise is all the more warranted and potentially fruitful.

Institute Events and Plans

As of this writing, the OCLC Institute has already completed several international seminars and scheduled several events for Fall 1997. A review of these events and other planning activities is presented below.

International OCLC Seminar. In June 1997, the Institute held a week-long seminar at the OCLC campus for a group of Brazilian academic library directors. The seminar, funded in part by the Andrew W. Mellon Foundation and the Fundação Getulio Vargas and Bibliodata Library Network, was entitled, "Information Technology Trends for the Global Library Community." Topics in the seminar ranged from trends in cataloging to telecommunications and the Internet 2 project. A full outline of the seminar is available through the OCLC Institute home page.

Moacyr Fioravante, director, Fundação Getulio Vargas, which is the administrative and operational center for the Brazilian Bibliodata Library Network, said of the Institute after the seminar, "Among the many important services that OCLC provides, I think that this initiative in education is going to be its most relevant contribution to the development of librarians and libraries with the competencies they need to cope with the emerging technologies, especially in less-developed countries." The seminar was very well received and the experience gained will be used as the basis for further such seminars.

Russian and Latvian Seminars. A need similar to that of Brazil exists in many parts of the world. For the most part, the need arises from the rapidity in the evolution of electronic knowledge. The pervasive adoption of digital technologies in the United States creates an advantage for U.S. knowledge industries compared to most of the rest of the world. This advantage is shared by OCLC member libraries. The problems faced by libraries in countries that were created with the dissolution of the USSR are different in degree and in kind from those in other parts of the world. Because they are suffering from chaotic economic conditions, they have fallen farther behind in the adoption of technology than many less-developed countries; because they have been closed societies for many decades, their preparation for participating in the global revolution in librarianship also needs foundation building. At the same time, they have a long tradition of support for libraries, particularly in the sciences, and a sophisticated grasp of the potential of technology to solve information problems. This unique combination of factors creates additional challenges for them and for anyone wishing to help them.

The seminars presented in Latvia and Russia were designed to open a dialogue, emphasizing the consequences of the new technology to librarianship and the new concepts that are arising in librarianship in response to it. Participants in both seminars were attentive and enthusiastic, with reasons for discouragement–primarily their lack of cash to purchase badly needed materials and equipment–balanced by the advantages of starting fresh.

Technology is helping make the world a smaller place. OCLC has multiple roles to play in this new world. One is to extend its services to include more of the world's libraries; another, and not very different, is to share with the world the concept of cooperative librarianship that helped establish OCLC.

Stated in simple terms, as the world moves toward a global village, it needs a global library.

Knowledge Access Management. This seminar, presented at OCLC in fall 1997, is subtitled "Tools and Concepts for Next-Generation Catalogers." Specifically designed for cataloging leaders, this seminar explores and advances the boundaries of digital cataloging practice in libraries through in-depth analysis of current practice, exploration of emerging technology applications, active discussion of cataloging futures, and distance learning and follow-on projects.

Technology Planning Seminar. This seminar, presented in Saratoga Springs, N.Y., in fall 1997, is entitled "Technology Planning in a Time of Change" and is designed for directors of medium to large academic libraries. Institute speakers will provide a strategic overview of technology trends and their impact on libraries. Facilitated round table discussion groups will allow attendees to investigate the implications of these trends for the allocation of library resources. Structured planning sessions and case studies will be incorporated into the seminar to help relate this information to the library environment.

Future Growth

As stated earlier, the OCLC Institute seeks to be responsive to demonstrated or expressed needs within the field, to exploit unique resources, and to leverage the multiplicative powers of partnerships. Crafting the exact mix and schedule of events will involve close consultation with U.S. Regional Networks, OCLC members and libraries generally, schools of library science, library professional organizations and other related groups. The resulting offerings, which will vary in terms of content, duration, location and cost, will nevertheless share the common goal of addressing current issues in library management and be intended for middle- and senior-level managers. Whatever the subject, however, the goal remains to provide opportunities for advanced education and knowledge exchange that will foster the evolution of libraries and library leaders.

While the focus of the institute in the near term will be on defining and presenting seminars and courses, three areas of possible long-term growth should be mentioned: consulting, distance learning and a visiting scholar program.

Opportunities may exist for the OCLC Institute to augment the consultative functions provided by U.S. Regional Networks and others. In the long term, as part of its teaching function, the OCLC Institute hopes to develop a capable staff that will be available to libraries as consultants.

A second area the institute plans to explore is distance learning. It is an attractive idea, mostly because of the (as yet unrealized) promise of unlimited leverage of technology in the presentation of courses. Just where it can be productive and where traditional classroom teaching and mentoring are required must be discovered through trial and error. It seems clear, however, that many teaching tasks can be accomplished through such media as Web-based exercises or CD-ROM-based, computer-assisted instruction. Active participation in this endeavor by the Institute can benefit the in-house training needs of OCLC, its member libraries, and U.S. Regional Networks, as well as being able to deliver course content from the Institute at reduced cost to participants.

There is also a role at OCLC for the Institute to provide positions for visiting scholars and internships to enrich both participants. OCLC's Office of Research program for visiting scholars has long been a valuable means of refreshing the pool of ideas and approaches available to OCLC. One hopes the program has benefited the visitors as well. A similar activity would be very worthwhile for the OCLC Institute, and in many respects less difficult to administer. The time required in residence by a visiting scholar to carry out a research activity of any significance is quite lengthy, usually a year. No such requirement is necessary for an Institute collaboration with visiting faculty or professionals from the field.

CONCLUSION

By many measures, the OCLC Institute is an idea whose time has come. Our world is being restructured at a dramatic rate by large-scale forces of change in the United States and increasingly outside the U.S. These forces so dwarf the concerns of libraries that they will often dictate the direction of library evolution. Though we are largely at their mercy, much can be done at the margins of these larger forces to define what libraries will become. Indeed, maneuvering in the margin may provide sufficient room for libraries to accomplish all that they desire.

Achieving the most effective definition of the library in the years to come must not be left to chance, and one major role of the OCLC Institute is to afford library professionals a forum for collaboratively, proactively and intentionally creating the world they desire. Two examples suffice to make this point, although many more are possible: electronic publication and the role of cataloging in the electronic library. In the next few years, changes in these areas will influence deeply what libraries become. It is doubtful that anyone can foresee the direction either will take. The library profession, through the energetic facilitation of agencies like the Institute, must help pilot the ship rather than observe from its deck chairs. Collaborative focus on directions and dangers and a constant eye on the home port are required.

OCLC is well positioned to collaborate with libraries in solving the problems posed by technology, to redefine the library profession, and to contribute to the evolution of its central concepts for the 21st century. The OCLC Institute is ready to assume an important role in this grand endeavor.

REFERENCES

1. Kevil, L. Hunter. 1996. "Continuing education and the reinvention of the library school." *Journal of Education for Library and Information Science* 37(2): 184-190.

2. Miller, Marilyn. 1996. "What to expect from library school graduates." *Information Technology and Libraries* 15(1): 45-47.

3. Ibid.

4. OCLC. 1994. *OCLC Articles of Incorporation*. October 1994, OCLC Online Computer Library Center, Inc. Article 3. Dublin, OH: OCLC.

OCLC's Office of Research:
Past, Present and Future

John V. Richardson, Jr.

In the field of library and information science, the OCLC Online Computer Library Center's Office of Research and Special Projects (OCLC OR) is one of the premier research organizations. Unlike library and information science faculty, its staff can devote 100 percent of their time to research. Yet OCLC OR's contributions, especially its role in technological innovation, are not as well known to the profession as they ought to be. For instance, no analytical or historical articles have been previously published about OCLC OR's work in the open literature.[1] Therefore, a historico-critical study of OCLC OR's development, present status and activities, and likely future direction would be an important contribution to advancing knowledge of its contributions. Such an examination is timely inasmuch as OCLC celebrated its thirtieth anniversary in 1997. Hence, the purpose of this article is: (1) to describe the historical development of the

Dr. John V. Richardson, Jr. is Associate Professor, Graduate School of Education and Information Studies, University of California, Los Angeles, and 1996/1997 OCLC Visiting Distinguished Scholar. At UCLA since 1978, he holds the PhD degree from Indiana University.

Direct all correspondence to: Dr. John V. Richardson, Jr., Graduate School of Education and Information Studies, Department of Library and Information Science, Box 951520, 204 GSE&IS Bldg., University of California, Los Angeles, Los Angeles, CA 90095-1520.

In particular, the author wishes to acknowledge Paula Julien, Records Management, OCLC Information Center and his colleagues, especially Bradley Watson for coordinating drafts of this manuscript, in the Office of Research where he spent his 1996/1997 academic year sabbatical as a Visiting Distinguished Scholar.

[Haworth co-indexing entry note]: "OCLC's Office of Research: Past, Present and Future." Richardson, John V., Jr. Co-published simultaneously in *Journal of Library Administration* (The Haworth Press, Inc.) Vol. 25, No. 4, 1998, pp. 201-238; and: *OCLC 1967-1997: Thirty Years of Furthering Access to the World's Information* (ed: K. Wayne Smith) The Haworth Press, Inc., 1998, pp. 201-238. Single or multiple copies of this article are available for a fee from The Haworth Document Delivery Service [1-800-342-9678, 9:00 a.m. - 5:00 p.m. (EST). E-mail address: getinfo@haworthpressinc.com].

Office within its institutional context; (2) to examine its present status, especially its current projects; and (3) to predict its likely future path. One might ask three key, guiding questions about OCLC's OR: Can they look to the past with pride? If one takes sober stock of the present, what would one find? And looking to the future, should one be optimistic? In fact, these are the questions that I propose to answer in this article because of their heuristic value to this investigation.

To structure and inform the following discussion, this article draws upon theoretical concepts such as STEPE, SWOT, and organizational theories from the management field.[2] Methodologically, this article employs several techniques including standard historiographical procedures (including work in the OCLC archives and Information Center), the case study method, and familiar ethnographic techniques (including personal interviews with current and former OR staff and directors as well as first-hand personal observations gleaned during an eleven-month sabbatical at OCLC).

BACKGROUND

By way of establishing a context, it is useful to know that OCLC is a tax exempt[3] organization of more than 1120 employees world-wide including Preservation Resources (formerly MAPS) in Bethlehem, Pennsylvania and Forest Press located in Lake Placid, New York. According to a recent annual report, the mission statement says that "OCLC is a nonprofit library computer service and research organization dedicated to the public purposes of furthering access to the world's information and reducing information costs."[4] Not long ago, its soon-to-retire[5] president, Dr. K. Wayne Smith, articulated four goals or strategies for OCLC during the next decade:

> The first goal is to integrate and enhance all OCLC core services by providing easy and seamless access to information. The second is to innovate by providing new, cost-effective, electronic alternatives such as archiving and new telecommunications technologies. The third is to internationalize by increasing global expansion and perspective. And, the fourth goal is to inform by adding educational services for the library and education communities, which we are already doing with the recently established OCLC Institute.[6]

Finally, Dr. Smith has also articulated OCLC's vision: "To provide seamless access to bibliographic, abstract and full-text information when and where people need it, at a price they can afford."[7]

Understandably, the Office of Research and Special Projects must operate within these four institutional givens (i.e., the organization's charter, mission, goal, and vision statements), if it is to remain viable. From a management perspective, such explicit statements can serve as potent motivating expressions for some employees.

Within OCLC, the Director of the Office of Research and Special Projects reports to the Executive Vice President and Chief Operating Officer, Donald J. Muccino. Special Projects includes 22 people, who work primarily in the distributed systems section. In terms of OR staffing, there are eight Research Scientists,[8] eleven Systems Analysts, seven Research Associates/Assistants, one occasional Visiting Distinguished Scholar, and two administrative support staff. They adopt a team approach to their research projects and come from diverse academic backgrounds including computer science, electrical engineering, industrial engineering, information transfer, library and information science, linguistics, natural resources, pharmacology, and physics. Almost all of the universities represented are in the Midwest, most typically Ohio State University. A Research Advisory Committee (RAC), which serves a three-year term, advises them on a semi-annual basis.[9] The current RAC is composed of Edward David (an industrial consultant and member of OCLC's Board of Trustees), Toni Carbo (University of Pittsburgh), Edward Fox (Virginia Polytechnic Institute and State University), and Bernie Hurley (University of California, Berkeley). The OR staff have written their own missional statement which says:

> [T]he OCLC Office of Research is to expand knowledge that advances OCLC's commitment to improved access to the world's information resources, whatever their form, substance, subject, language or location.[10]

Furthermore, "This mission is pursued through the integrated employment of the computer, library, and information sciences in research activities such as performing experiments, building prototypes, advancing standards, undertaking studies, and participating in research collaborations."[11]

The management of innovation is demanding. Since January 1974, eight Directors have led the Office of Research (see Table 1), which is an average of one new director every 3.6 years. During Frederick G. Kilgour's founding presidency, James E. Rush headed up the Research and Development Group. However, W. David Penniman gets credit for "creat[ing] the research organization at OCLC"[12] during his tenure as anager of the Research Department during the late 1970s. From January 1981 to June 1983, as Manager of the Department and then Director of

TABLE 1. Directors of the Office of Research and Special Projects, 1974-date

---

1. James E. Rush, January 1974-1975; March 1980-January 1981

2. W. David Penniman, Research Manager, February 1978-December 1979; Vice President of Research and Planning, 1982-1984

3. Neal K. Kaske, January 1981-July 1983

4. Thomas B. Hickey, Acting, July 1983-June 1984; Co-Acting, June 1993-May 1994

5. Michael J. McGill, July 1984-July 1986

6. Martin Dillon, July 1986-1993

7. Edward T. O'Neill, Co-Acting, June 1993-May 1994

8. Terry R. Noreault, May 1994-date

SOURCE: OCLC Online Computer Library Center, Inc. Corporate Archives

Office of Research, Neal Kaske "led a team that started building a knowledge base on the use made of online public access catalogs in libraries with significant outside funding from CLR and NSF, and by cooperatively working with RLG."[13] Michael J. McGill served as Acting Director of the Office from July 1984 to July 1986. McGill formalized many of the present activities such as a research advisory panel, the external relations program, a research intelligence effort, a technology assessment activity, educational activities, and the publication of research news.[14] The longest-serving director to date has been Martin Dillon (1986-1994). When asked about his accomplishments, Dillon replied: "to get OR to focus on OCLC member problems and not general research. Some specific results: usability lab, authority service, collections analysis CD, electronic Dewey, [and] Internet research that led to Intercat and Netfirst."[15] The current director of Research is Terry Noreault who took office in May 1994; as for his accomplishments, he believes that OR had "embraced web technologies and developed a vigorous research program exploring their application to libraries."[16]

From a historical perspective, four OR projects stand out as truly innovative. (An Appendix to this article contains a chronology of people, projects and libraries involved in OR since 1985.) The first project is a late 1970s videotext effort called Channel 2000, a two-way cable television delivery of information into a couple of hundred Columbus area households. Some might even argue that the Department of Research was established within OCLC's Office of Planning and Research to provide such home delivery of library services (HDLS). By way of background, OCLC's first president, Frederick G. Kilgour, observed the British Prestel/ Viewdata and presciently observed that OCLC could be doing much more in this area. The Channel 2000 ViewTel videotex was field-tested[17] for a 90-day period in late 1980 by its end users. They could access the Public Library of Columbus and Franklin County's library catalog and have books delivered via mail, consult the full-text of articles from *The Academic American Encyclopedia* online, check the local community calendar, and even retrieve limited banking data from Banc One and pay bills.[18] The innovative decoder keypad had several user-friendly keys labeled "Oops," "Get," and "Do It."[19] Ultimately, the project was not fruitful, in part because its marketing researchers were ahead of demand for such services, but it does sound a lot like today's WebTV.

The inability to display bibliographic information effectively from catalog cards has been a persistent concern in OR. In the late 1970s, only uppercase characters were used for display on most computer screens or printouts. Besides the need for lowercase, additional typographic issues (such as accents, scientific formula, and non-roman characters) immediately consume one's attention. Tom Hickey labored for ten years on various aspects of this problem. Much of what he learned came as a result of GRAPH-TEXT,[20] a prototype electronic delivery system that allowed libraries to print out journal articles on demand. Using typesetting tapes from the American Chemical Society, Elsevier, Scientific American, and the World Book Company, he scanned this information into the computer and used Donald Knuth's TEX system for display purposes. The system ran on an AT-class IBM computer, using a CD-ROM disk to store the reformatted images and text. Using a networked printer, royalties could be tracked as well. Interestingly, many users changed their attitudes toward these charges; they believed they owned the information and did not want to pay per-page charges. In any event, when this project ended in the late 1980s,[21] electronic publishing, notably OCLC's Electronic Journals Online program, was a well-established concept.

Next, Ed O'Neill's contribution to maintaining and enhancing the database quality must be discussed. In 1978/79, O'Neill joined OR as a Visiting Distinguished Scholar to develop an algorithm for subject access. However, he quickly noticed that the menu display of these headings revealed many errors, mostly misspellings.[22] In June 1983, he came back as a Research Scientist to continue working on a subject access prototype, but again got caught up in error correction. By 1985/86 there was widespread concern in the profession about dirty[23] databases. If true for OCLC, such a situation could have caused lower cataloging productivity and in the worst case, a jumping of ship to WLN or RLIN. For sure, OCLC quality control staff were getting error reports in excess of their capacity to deal with them and finally had to give priority to those that affected search keys. Ultimately, as many as one million duplicate records have been deleted in order to maintain the high standards expected of OCLC's WorldCat.[24]

Finally, there is OR's continuing desire to provide information to the user, especially on the desktop computer, with the least effort. Stu Weibel's contribution in the early 1990s was the Chemical Online Retrieval Experiment project (CORE), one of the first large-scale digital library projects which preceded the heavily-funded NSF/NASA/ARPA Digital Library Initiative by five years.[25] CORE's goal was to render much of a discipline's current literature into SGML, an electronic format, so that scholars could search, browse, read and print formulae, figures, and text from their workstations. OCLC decided to work with the American Chemical Society and scan four years' worth of articles from 20 of their scholarly journals (about 400,000 pages taking 10 gigabytes of storage space). User studies indicate that the project was popular with chemists who appreciated the enhanced search capabilities, liked the browsing of thumbnail versions of the figures, and the ability to organize their own display screens.

CURRENT SITUATION

In 1996, the most recent year for which data is available, OCLC spent $14 million company-wide in research and development (R&D).[26] Although there has not been double-digit growth, OR works within a good, if not strong, economic environment where OCLC's gross and net revenues have been up 17 out of 19 years and 10 out of 12 years respectively. And, whether one looks at gross or net revenue since 1978, OCLC commits an average of nine percent to R&D per year. To put this figure in perspective, one might compare it to six percent for Xerox Parc (over the period of 1993-95) or 36 percent for SAS Institute (over the period 1987-95).

Some of these funds are committed to external and collaborative research, notably the Library and Information Science Research Grant Program (LISRG) which provides two or three yearly $10,000 grants to library and information science educators and professionals.[27] In addition, they have offered a Visiting Distinguished Scholar (VDS) program which has invited such individuals as Abraham Bookstein, Martin Dillon, Karen Drabensott, Fran Miksa, Edward O'Neill, Elaine Svenonius, and Terry

Noreault to come to OCLC for a period of time; obviously, several VDSers have stayed on. The Postdoctoral Fellowship program has supported a variety of individuals including Diane Vizine-Goetz, Chandra Prabha, and Mike Prasse, who were retained by OCLC, too. Finally, there is the Distinguished Seminar series, established in 1978, which brings noted individuals to speak to OCLC staff about pressing matters.[28]

In characterizing the recent work in library and information science one could classify it along the following lines: the needs of libraries (which in the 1970s focused on library settings and then in the 1980s on library services) and non-library settings (especially electronic resources in the 1990s). Ignoring type-of-library studies, OR has clearly contributed to understanding library services better. In the broad context of preservation, especially selection of materials, note OR's work on holdings and sources,[29] collection development analysis,[30] and deterioration of library materials.[31] On the access side of the house, cataloging and classification studies predominate; for example, time and work flow,[32] Cataloger's Assistant,[33] OPACS,[34] Chinese records,[35] neural networks,[36] Library of Congress Subject Headings,[37] Dewey call numbers,[38] and Dewey 2000.[39] Back-of-the book indexing[40] has been studied. Nor have information retrieval,[41] interlibrary loan,[42] and resource sharing[43] been overlooked.

One of the most promising efforts, with both short and long-term payoffs, is WordSmith.[44] Jean Godby is drawing upon computational linguistic techniques to create more useful meta-level indexes, such as online browseable thesauri rather than single term word count indexes, to html pages. The short-term benefits are already demonstrable on an internal OR collection of web pages while the long-term benefits should include automatic mining of databases for facts and data as well as automatic subject heading assignments.

More recently, the needs of users have come to the forefront and much LIS work has shifted to user-friendly interfaces, a self-service orientation, and point of service. Likewise, OR shifted its attention to, for example, user interface efforts,[45] browsing issues[46] or business research and planning.[47] Now in the late 1990s, with technological advances in electronic access, non-library settings have taken over. So, OR has looked into electronic publishing (i.e., Fred, Guidon, and Kilroy research projects)[48] and resource description on the Worldwide Web.[49]

Following OCLC's 1991 strategic planning initiative,[50] one could ask how OR: (1) enhances the existing base of products and services and adds new products and services; (2) maintains the world-class database of bibliographic information; and (3) moves beyond bibliography to become a world-class provider of reference services, including full-text electronic information? Strictly speaking, enhancement of existing products is development work and not OR's responsibility per se, nonetheless it has provided enhancements in subject searching in OCLC's existing products. Several projects in OR, such as cataloging and classification research, help maintain existing OCLC products. In the innovative category, one must cite FirstSearch, Electronic Journals Online, Search CD450, the promising resource description framework of metadata[51] and the Platform for Internet Content Selection (PICS) work[52] as well as OR's electronic reference services work.[53] Taking the world-class concept a bit further, OCLC's WorldCat is certainly the most comprehensive database of its kind and one of the top two or three most important bibliographic databases anywhere, but there are strong competitors such as Elsevier, Lexis/Nexis, and the Web itself.

When asked to name their own successful projects, some OR staff replied: (1) FirstSearch; (2) GRAPH-TEXT; (3) duplicate detection and deletion; (4) PURL, Scorpion, and Fred; and (5) Dublin Core/PICS/ Resource Description Framework.[54] And, if one wonders why they considered these projects to be successful, one only need look at: (1) the quality of the people involved; (2) the years of expertise involved; (3) the good idea which started it; and (4) the team approach to problem solving that has allowed projects to transition from projects to products.

THE FUTURE

Few would disagree that the LIS environment is changing; hence, there are new challenges and alternative service providers. Organizational theory, drawing upon thinking in biology and ecology, argues that a group's survival is dependent upon its fit within a particular niche as well as its ability to evolve. One challenge is the need to re-examine end-user requirements and adopt a more user-centered system design philosophy. In the near future, for instance, we may have intelligent agents and e-cash on the Worldwide Web. Conceivably, we may not even pay for information in the future, if Microsoft purchased all of the information industry, which it could do out of current revenue streams alone. In the near term, though, Ameritech is one of the viable alternative service providers.[55] Other political and social threats to OR's long-term survival include: changes in top management at OCLC; the number of catalogers is declining and their mean age is increasing;[56] the shifting focus on the library from a physical to virtual place; the fact that libraries are tax-supported institutions and society, for the moment, prefers lower taxes;[57] and other service providers, such as DRA's Library2000 project, which has interesting solutions to sharing cataloging records.

OR has numerous opportunities to keep OCLC on the leading edge, for instance: (1) it could examine the OCLC product architecture to establish a common platform much like Black and Decker did in the 1970s or Chrysler and the entire automotive industry did in the 1980s, in order to respond to changing market needs and the need to lower costs;[58] and (2) OR could capitalize on the fact that "computing is cheaper and easier, telecommunications is cheaper and easier, there is more free information, and more electronic information."[59] While the 35 million-record[60] database (WorldCat, the Online Union Catalog) is a fabulous repository that is the basis for almost all of OCLC's information products, a common platform could shorten the long development cycle and derivative projects could come to market much sooner. A shared access platform is only logical.

The U.S. chemical industry's document *Technology Vision 2020* asserts that "over the next 25 years the chemical industry must improve efficiency in the use of raw materials and energy, play a leadership role in balancing environmental and economic considerations, and aggressively commit to long-term investment in research. With this guidance, the industry will thrive and continue to be a responsible neighbor in the global community, protecting environmental quality and economic well-being while promoting our quality of life."[61] Substituting "information" for chemical in the above quotation makes interesting reading.

The Next Steps in Understanding OR

In order to gain an additional deeper understanding of the Office of Research, one might undertake three studies: (1) personality types and their role in team research; (2) influence of birth order and creativity; and (3) the analysis of social interactions. Suppose for instance, the Myers-Briggs-Type Indicator, a widely used personality inventory, revealed that OR staff were predominately designers (INTPs, meaning introvert-intuition-thinking-perceiving types) and entailers (INTJs, meaning introvert-intuition-thinking-judging types). Would it be appropriate to seek out the opposite types such as ESFJs (extrovert-sensing-feeling-judging types) or ESFPs (meaning extrovert-sensing-feeling-perceiving types)?[62] Similarly, there is a body of research that suggests openness to scientific innovation can be influenced by numerous factors including birth order.[63] Again, suppose most OR staff members were last-born individuals, what implications are there for continued technological innovation?[63] Finally, one could construct a social network model (a.k.a. sociogram) of the OR workplace to understand better inter-personal communication.

CONCLUSION

In summary, I believe that the OR can look to the past with a measure of pride. It has made several significant technological innovations as described above. Taking sober stock of the present, I believe that OR is an open, flexible and cooperative environment that is committed to solving significant problems in library and information science. Being responsive to their environment, OR has been willing to change its research agenda as needed, but it may still need to communicate better with end-users to determine requirements by working through OCLC's marketing department. I know OR values innovation. Finally, I do not believe it is an exaggeration to say that OCLC's future is the Office of Research. If they find new blood (to achieve a better gender and ethnic balance as well as people with experience or degrees from universities on a broad, international basis) for its staffing and achieve continuity of leadership at the Director level which is necessary to maintain this innovative group culture, I believe that OCLC's Office of Research can look to the future with optimism and determination.

NOTES

1. Although a good primary source of information is their internal *Annual Review of OCLC Research*, published annually since 1986.

2. Strategic planning occurs within a Social, Technical, Economic, Political and Ecological (STEPE) context. SWOT stands for Strengths, Weaknesses, Opportunities, and Threats. Both analyses were applied during "Research & Reflection: The 1997 Office of Research Retreat" at Burr Oak Lodge, Ohio to assess future directions.

3. According to the Internal Revenue Service, a tax exempt organization includes "Corporations, and any community chest, fund, or foundation, organized and operated exclusively for religious, charitable, scientific, testing for public safety, literary, or educational purposes, or to foster national or international amateur sports competition (but only if no part of its activities involve the provision of athletic facilities or equipment), or for the prevention of cruelty to children or animals, no part of the net earnings of which inures to the benefit of any private share-holder or individual, no substantial part of the activities of which is carrying on propaganda, or otherwise attempting, to influence legislation (except as otherwise provided in subsection (h)), and which does not participate in, or intervene in (including the publishing or distributing of statements), any political campaign on behalf of (or in opposition to) any candidate for public office" from section 501(c)(3) of the *Internal Revenue Code of 1986*.

4. *OCLC. 1996. OCLC Annual Report 1995/96* (Dublin, OH: OCLC Online Computer Library Center, Inc.): 1. According to its *Articles of Incorporation* (of

1981 and 1977, but paraphrasing and expanding 5 July 1967), "The purpose or purposes for which this Corporation is formed are to establish, maintain and operate a computerized library network and to promote the evolution of library use, of libraries themselves, and of librarianship, and to provide processes and products for the benefit of library users and libraries, including such objectives as increasing availability of library resources to individual library patrons and reducing the rate of rise of library per-unit costs, all for the fundamental public purpose of furthering ease of access to and use of the ever-expanding body of world-wide scientific, literary and educational knowledge and information."

5. Smith, K. Wayne. 1997. "Business as Usual." *OCLC Newsletter* (September/October) No. 229: 3.

6. OCLC. 1997. *Beyond 2000: A Summary of OCLC's Strategic Plan* (Dublin, OH: OCLC Online Computer Library Center, Inc.): 1. Dr. Smith presented these four goals publicly in a slightly different version with a gloss at the Research Library Directors Conference in March 1997.

7. OCLC. 1996. *1995/96 Annual Report*: 3.

8. In the beginning there were only three titles, not unlike academe: Assistant Research Scientist, Research Scientist and Senior Research Scientist; over time, there has been some title inflation with the creation of two more titles: Chief and Consulting Research Scientist series.

9. Founded in 1984, eighteen people (three of whom were women) have served as RAC members, primarily from university settings; see OR's "Research Advisory Committee, Collective List, Past Members," undated.

10. Close paraphrase from the *Annual Review of OCLC Research 1995*. 1996. (Dublin, OH: OCLC Online Computer Library Center, Inc.): cover.

11. See *http://www.oclc.org:5047/oclc/research/rspd/rspd_page.html*

12. Personal interview with David Penniman, Spring 1997.

13. Personal interview with Neal Kaske, Spring 1997.

14. In particular, McGill hired Jeffrey Katzer of Syracuse University to serve as a consultant to create the "Development Plan for the OCLC Office of Research,"16 July 1984. That same year, Katzer also led the first of many OR retreats; the purpose of the first retreat on 12-13 November at Ohio State University's Fawcett Center was "to establish a prioritization of research areas. The goal is to define categories of research areas . . ."(Mike McGill to OR Staff, 26 October 1984 memorandum). Personal interview with Mike McGill, 8 November 1997.

15. Personal interview with Martin Dillon, Spring 1997.

16. Personal interview with Terry Noreault, Spring and 8 November 1997.

17. Tom Harnish, the HDLS Program Manager, argued that its users would only settle for the best that they had seen elsewhere. An Ohio State University doctoral dissertation by William T. Bolton Jr. entitled "The Perception and Potential Adoption of Channel 2000: Implications for Diffusion Theory and Videotex Technology" (1981) found that the user's attitude depended upon their prior experience with information systems–novices loved it while more sophisticated users expected what they were already familiar with in their labs.

18. Channel 2000 is not well covered in the research literature while QUBE, the contemporaneous Warner-Amex effort in Columbus, Ohio, is more so. See Noll, A. Michael. 1995. *Highway of Dreams: A Critical Appraisal of the Information Superhighway* (Los Angeles: USC Bookstore Custom Pub.); Greenberger, Martin. 1985. *Electronic Publishing Plus: Media for a Technological Future* (White Plains, NY: Knowledge Industry Publications, Inc.); and Rogers, Everett M. 1986. *Communication Technology: The New Media in Society* (New York: Free Press). While the HDLS key players are still available, someone should examine this topic more closely.

19. The Channel 2000 effort did result in the first two of OCLC's five patents: 4,451,701 Viewdata System and Apparatus,"(Mark Bendig, inventor; 29 May 1984) and 4,581,484, "Audio-Enhanced Videotex System" (Mark Bendig, inventor; 8 April 1986).

20. OCLC's Video Communications Program's first near production quality VHS videotape was a ten-minute demonstration by Thomas Hickey entitled "GRAPH-TEXT" on 8 January 1986.

21. See Hickey, Thomas B. Hickey. 1989. "Using SGML and TEX for an Interactive Chemical Encyclopedia." *National Online Meeting: Proceedings of the Tenth National Online Meeting, New York, 9-11 May 1989*, compiled by Carol Nixon and Lauree Padgett (Medford, NJ: Learned Information): 187-95.

22. See his humorously entitled talk, " 'Addrdsses, Elctures, Esssays *[sic]*' and other Variant Subject Headings," with Anna E. Lantz and Diane Vizine-Goetz in *Proceedings of the Third National Conference of the Association of College and Research Libraries* (Chicago: American Library Association, 1984). In addition, at least two dissertations resulted from this work: Aluri, Rao. 1981. "Subject Access to Catalog Records in Large Bibliographic Data Bases." Ph.D. Dissertation, SUNY at Buffalo, and Vizine-Goetz, Diana. 1983. "A Computer Algorithm for Correcting Spelling and Typographic Errors in Subject Headings." Ph.D. Dissertation, Case Western Reserve University.

23. For example at one point, catalogers were using OCLC to share an apple-sauce cake recipe via a MARC-formatted record.

24. A good summary of the situation appears in O'Neill, Edward T. and Diane Vizine-Goetz. 1988. "Quality Control and Online Systems." *Annual Review of Information Science and Technology* (Netherlands: Elsevier Science Publications): 125-156.

25. Entlich, Richard, Lorrin Garson, Michael Lesk, Lorraine Normore, Jan Olsen, and Stu Weibel. 1997. "Making a Digital Library: The Contents of the CORE Project." *ACM Transactions on Information Systems* 15 (April): 103-23.

26. More precisely, Dr. Smith estimates that OCLC spends $5 million a year on applied research; see Smith, K. Wayne. 1997. "OCLC Research Helps Libraries Build for the Future." *OCLC Newsletter* (January/February) No. 225: 3. Obviously, OR's budget is something less than this figure.

27. Since 1985, OR has made 74 grants totaling more than $493,827 plus equipment; see "Office of Research Grant Awards, 1985-Present," Fall 1997.

28. See OR's "Distinguished Seminar Series Speaker List by Date," revised 26 March 1997, which lists 75 speakers.

29. Serebnick, Judith. 1992. "Selection and Holdings of Small Publishers' Books in OCLC Libraries: A Study of the Influence of Reviews, Publishers, and Vendors." *Library Quarterly* 62 (July): 259-94.

30. O'Neill, Edward T. 1978. "The Effect of Demand Level on the Optimal Size of Journal Collections." *Collection Management* 2 (Fall): 205-216.

31. O'Neill, Edward T. and Wesley L. Boomgaarden. 1996. "Book Deterioration and Loss: Magnitude and Characteristics in Ohio Libraries." *Library Resources and Technical Services* 39: 395-408.

32. Prabha, Chandra. 1989. "Cataloging Time and Workflow Studies." *Annual Review of OCLC Research: July 1988-June 1989*. Dublin, OH: OCLC Online Computer Library Center, Inc.: 9-11 and Prabha, Chandra. 1992. "Costs, Workflows and Usage Data for Interlibrary Loan and Document Delivery." *Annual Review of OCLC Research July 1991-June 1992*. Dublin, OH: OCLC Online Computer Library Center, Inc.: 18-21.

33. Vizine-Goetz, Diane. 1989. "Catalogers Assistant." *Annual Review of OCLC Research July 1988-June 1989*. Dublin, OH: OCLC Online Computer Library Center, Inc.: 8-9 and Vizine-Goetz, Diane. 1991. "Cataloging Productivity Tools." *Annual Review of OCLC Research July 1990-June 1991*. Dublin, OH: OCLC Online Computer Library Center, Inc.: 8-10.

34. Belkin, Nicholas and Tefko Saracevic. 1992. "Design Principles for Third Generation Online Public Access Catalogs." *Annual Review of OCLC Research July 1991-June 1992*. Dublin, OH: OCLC Online Computer Library Center, Inc.: 43-45.

35. Rasmussen, Edie and Marcia Lei Zeng. 1992. "The Quality of Chinese Records in the OCLC Database." *Annual Review of OCLC Research July 1991-June 1992*. Dublin, OH: OCLC Online Computer Library Center, Inc.: 58-60.

36. Weibel, Stuart. 1989. "Applying Neural Networks to Classification Problems." *Annual Review of OCLC Research July 1988-June 1989*. Dublin, OH: OCLC Online Computer Library Center, Inc.: 3-4.

37. Chan, Lois and Diane Vizine-Goetz. 1996. "Feasibility of a Computer-generated Subject Validation File Based on Frequency of Occurrence of Assigned LC Subject Headings." *Annual Review of OCLC Research 1995*. Dublin, OH: OCLC Online Computer Library Center, Inc.: 46-52.

38. O'Neill, Edward T., Brian F. Lavoie, Jeffrey A. Young and Patrick D. McClain. 1997. "Four-Figure Cutter Tables." *Annual Review of OCLC Research 1996*. Dublin, OH: OCLC Online Computer Library Center, Inc.: 1-18.

39. Vizine-Goetz, Diane and Joan S. Mitchell. 1996. "Dewey 2000." *Annual Review of OCLC Research 1995*. Dublin, OH: OCLC Online Computer Library Center, Inc.: 16-19.

40. Liddy, Elizabeth D. 1992. "The Art of Back-of-the-Book Indexes." *Annual Review of OCLC Research 1991-1992*. Dublin, OH: OCLC Online Computer Library Center, Inc.: 34-36.

41. Prabha, Chandra. 1991. "The Large Retrieval Phenomenon." *Advances in Library Automation and Networking* Vol. 4. Edited by Joe A. Hewitt (Greenwich, CT: JAI Press): 55-92.

42. Yu, Clement and Chengjie Luo. 1992. "Implementation and Performance Evaluation of an Image Decompression Algorithm." *Annual Review of OCLC Research 1991-1992*. Dublin, OH: OCLC Online Computer Library Center, Inc.: 46-47.

43. Prabha, Chandra and John E. Ogden. 1994. "Recent Trends in Academic Library Materials Expenditures." *Library Trends* 42 (Winter): 499-513 and Prabha, Chandra and Elisabeth Marsh. 1997. "Commercial Development Suppliers: How Many of the ILL/DD Periodical Requests Can They Fulfill?" *Library Trends* 45 (Winter): 551-568.

44. See the WordSmith home page on OCLC's intracat at *http://orc/ WordSmith/wshome.html*

45. Dillon, Martin, ed. 1991. *Interfaces for Information Retrieval and Online Systems* (Westport, CT: Greenwood Press) and Lindeman, Martha J. 1989. "Interface Styles from an Interface Designer's Perspective." *Journal of the American Society for Information Science* 15 (April/May): 16-17 as well as Ben Shneiderman.

46. Kwasnik, Barbara H. 1992. "The Functional Components of Browsing." *Annual Review of OCLC Research 1991-1992*. Dublin, OH: OCLC Online Computer Library Center, Inc.: 53-56.

47. Crook, Mark A. 1996. "Business-oriented Research and Planning." *Annual Review of OCLC Research 1995*. Dublin, OH: OCLC Online Computer Library Center, Inc.: 2-3.

48. Fausey, John R. and Keith E. Shafer. 1996. "World Wide Web Access to FRED." *Annual Review of OCLC Research 1995*. Dublin, OH: OCLC Online Computer Library Center, Inc.: 20-22 and Hickey, Thomas J. 1996. "Guidon Web: Applying Java to Scholarly Electronic Journals." *Annual Review of OCLC Research 1995*. Dublin, OH: OCLC Online Computer Library Center, Inc.: 22-25 and Keith E. Shafer. 1997. "Kilroy: An Internet Research Project." *Annual Review of OCLC Research 1996*. Dublin, OH: OCLC Online Computer Library Center, Inc.: 44-45.

49. Shafer, Keith E. 1997. "Automatic Subject Assignment via the Scorpion System." *Annual Review of OCLC Research 1996*. Dublin, OH: OCLC Online Computer Library Center, Inc.: 20-21.

50. Paraphrasing "Strategic Overview, Vision: 1995-2000" from *Journey to the 21st Century: A Summary of OCLC's Strategic Plan*. 1991. Dublin, OH: OCLC Online Computer Library Center, Inc.: 11.

51. Forthcoming: Miller, Eric. "The World Wide Web Consortium's Resource Description Framework." *Annual Review of OCLC Research 1997*. Dublin, OH: OCLC Online Computer Library Center, Inc.

52. Weibel, Stuart and Eric Miller. 1997. "Cataloging Syntax and Public Policy Meet in PICS." *OCLC Newsletter* (May/June) No. 227: 28-29.

53. For first-hand demonstration, try *http://purl.oclc.org/net/Question_Master* or read John V. Richardson Jr., "Question Master: An Evaluation of a Web-based Decision-Support System for Use in Reference Environments." 1998. *College and Research Libraries* 59 (January): in press.

54. Based on small-group discussions during "Research and Reflection: The 1997 Office of Research Retreat" at Burr Oak Lodge, Ohio on 12-13 June 1997.

55. See Ameritech's AmLibs' corporate vision and three strategies on the Web at *http://www.ameritech.com/news/international/library.html*

56. Consider the following as a potential harbinger of change: there are no catalogers per se at the University of California, Berkeley.

57. Having said that, though, local library tax issues pass at a high rate.

58. See Meyer, Marc H. and Michael H. Zack. 1996. "The Design and Development of Information Products." *Sloan Management Review* 37 (Spring): 43–59.

59. Hickey, Thomas J. 1997. "Review of Research." 14 March.

60. As of 30 June 1997.

61. *http://208.209.231.7/pafgen/washalrt/wa97/wa012197.htm*

62. See Hirsch, Sandra K. 1991. *Using the Myers-Briggs Type Indicator in Organizations*, 2nd ed. (Palo Alto, CA: Consulting Psychologists Press) and Scherdin, Mary J. *Discovering Librarians: Profiles of a Profession* 1994. (Chicago: American Library Association), especially section III. For a contrarian view, read Blinkhorn, Steve and Charles Johnson. 1990. "The Insignificance of Personality Testing," *Nature* 348 (20/27 December): 671-72.

63. (New York: Pantheon Books, 1996).

APPENDIX

RESEARCH AT OCLC: PROMOTING THE EVOLUTION OF LIBRARIES, OF LIBRARY USE AND OF LIBRARIANSHIP

Here is a chronology of people, projects and libraries involved in the OCLC Office of Research since 1985.

1985/86

OCLC Research Projects

"Advanced Interface Design for Library Retrieval Systems," Martin Dillon

"Automated Title Page Cataloging," Stuart L. Weibel

"Class Dispersion between the LC Classification and the DDC," Diane Vizine-Goetz

"Collection Analysis," Edward T. O'Neill

"CONSER Abstracting and Indexing Title Overlap," John E. Tolle

"Dewey Decimal Classification Online," Karen Markey

"Display Formats," John E. Tolle

"Electronic Information Delivery Online System (EIDOS)," Betsy N. Kiser

"Graph-Text," Thomas B. Hickey

"Nonfiction Book Use by Public Library Users," Chandra G. Prabha

"OCLC CD-ROM Retrieval System," Terry R. Noreault

"OCLC Database Use Analysis," Brigitte L. Kenney

"Subject Access," Edward T. O'Neill

External and Collaborative Research

"American Fiction Project," Geoffrey D. Smith, Robert A. Tibbetts, William J. Crowe, Edward T. O'Neill, Diane Vizine-Goetz

Applied Information Technologies Research Center

MIT Media Laboratory

VOCAT Project

Distinguished Seminar Series

"Databases: Dinosaurs to Compact Discs," M. Lynn Neufeld

"The Generation of Complex Content Descriptions for Document Identification," Gerard Salton and Joe Fagan

"Preservation Administration in Research Libraries: Making the Past Accessible to the Future," Wesley L. Boomgaarden

"Optical Disk Technology and Library Needs," Joseph W. Price

"Electronic Information Handling Technologies: Preservation Issues," Charles M. Dollars

"Cataloging for the Electronic Union Catalog," Michael Gorman

"The Use of Machine-Readable Databases in Technological and Social Forecasting," F. W. Lancaster

Research Advisory Committee

Robert M. Hayes, Dean, Graduate School of Library and Information Science, University of California, Los Angeles

Michael E. Lesk, Manager, Computer Science Research Division, Bell Communication Research

Brian J. Perry, Director, Research and Development Department, British Library

Douglas E. Van Houweling, Vice Provost for Information Technology, University of Michigan

Visiting Scholars

Martin Dillon, Professor, Library Science, University of North Carolina, Chapel Hill

Terry R. Noreault, Assistant Professor, Information Science, University of Pittsburgh

1986/87

OCLC Research Projects

"Advanced Interface Management," Martin Dillon

"Applying Measures of Dispersion to the Library of Congress and Dewey Decimal Classification Systems," Diane Vizine-Goetz

"Automated Title Page Cataloging," Stuart L. Weibel

"Collection Analysis System," Mark A. Crook

"Comparative Classification," Francis L. Miksa

"Database Quality," Edward T. O'Neill

"Graph-Text," Thomas B. Hickey

"Library of Congress Class M Subset: Music," Jeanette M. Drone

"Nonfiction Book Use by Academic Library Users," Chandra G. Prabha

"Online Union Catalog Subsetting Analysis," John A. Bunge

External and Collaborative Research

Applied Information Technologies Research Center

"Automatic Syntax-based Phrase Construction for Content Analysis in Document Retrieval," Gerard Salton

"Increasing the Accessibility of Library of Congress Subject Headings in Online Bibliographic Systems," Karen Markey and Diane Vizine-Goetz

"Media Laboratory," Nicholas Negroponte

"Name-Authority Project," Jerry D. Saye

"Study Group on the Structure of Electronic Text," Thomas J. Michalak and Dana S. Scott

"Term Weighting in Document Retrieval," Clement T. Yu

"Vocabularies of Criticism and Theory," Ralph Cohen and James Sosnoski

Library and Information Science Research Grants

"Assessing Access to Alternative Press Publications: Women's Press Titles in the OCLC Online Union Catalog," Suzanne Hildenbrand

"Dynamics of the OCLC Online Union Catalog," Debra Shaw

"Holdings as a Measure of Journal Value," Danny P. Wallace

"Studies in Automated Cataloging," Elaine Svenonius

"Tables of Contents in Online Public Access Catalogs," Mark T. Kinnucan

"Variations in Subject Cataloging in Non-Library of Congress Cataloging Records," Lois Mai Chan

Distinguished Seminar Series

"Feedback Mechanisms in Information Retrieval," Abraham Bookstein

"Information Retrieval Research: Interface Comparison, Database Selection, and Transparent Systems," Martha E. Williams

"Evaluating the Impact of Implementing an Integrated Automated Library System," Jose-Marie Griffiths

"Capturing Concepts with Data Structures," Dana S. Scott

"Novel Aspects of Ada," Narain H. Gehani

"The Vanishing Library Catalog: Access, Bibliography, and Technology," Michael Buckland

"Project Quartet," Brian Shackel

"The Work and the Work Record in Cataloging," Patrick Wilson

Research Advisory Committee Members

Robert M. Hayes, Dean, Graduate School of Library and Information Science, University of California, Los Angeles

Michael E. Lesk, Manager, Computer Science Research Division

Brian Perry, Director, British Library, London

Douglas E. Van Houweling, The University of Michigan, Ann Arbor

Visiting Scholar

Francis L. Miksa, Professor, Library and Information Science, University of Texas at Austin

1987/88

OCLC Research Projects

"Advanced Interface Management," Martin Dillon and Martha Gordon Lindeman

"Automated Document Structure Analysis," Stuart L. Weibel

"Clustering Equivalent Bibliographic Records," Elaine Svenonius

"Collection Analysis," Edward T. O'Neill

"Collection Analysis System," David J. Stephens

"Connectionist Models of Computation," Stuart L. Weibel

"Database Quality," Edward T. O'Neill

"Document Facsimile Transmission Studies," John C. Handley

"Duplicate Detection and the 'Species Problem,' " John A. Bunge

"Graph-Text," Thomas B. Hickey

"Information Display," Thomas B. Hickey

"Information Services Project," Mark A. Crook

"Library of Congress Class M Subset: Music," Jeanette M. Drone

"Managing Large Retrievals," Chandra G. Prabha

"Nonfiction Book Use," Chandra G. Prabha

"Scholars Cross-Reference System," Paul B. Kantor

"Selecting Bibliographic Records," John A. Bunge

External and Collaborative Research

"Automatic Phrase Construction for the Representation of Text Content," Gerard Salton

"Extensions to the Advanced Interface Management Project," Niall Teskey

"Increasing the Accessibility of Library of Congress Subject Headings in Online Bibliographic Systems," Karen Markey

"Latvian Bibliographic Records in the Online Union Catalog," Inese Auzina Smith

"Mercury: An Electronic Library," William Y. Arms, Mark H. Kibbey, Thomas J. Michalak, James H. Morris, Dana S. Scott, Marvin A. Sirbu, Martin Dillon, and Michael J. McGill

"Term Weighting in Document Retrieval," Clement T. Yu and Hirotaka Mizuno

Library and Information Science Research Grants

"Analytical Study of Bibliographic Data on a Title Page," Billie Grace

"Applying the Revised MARC Format for Three-dimensional Objects in Museums," Esther G. Bierbaum

"Converting English Subject Headings into Spanish," Emilia Bernal-Rosa

"Evaluating Subject Collections," Howard D. White

"Measurement of Subject Scatter in the Superintendent of Documents Classification," Lee Shiflett

"Subject Representations in Monographic Records," Pamela Reekes McKirdy

"Variations in Personal and Corporate Names in the OCLC Online Union Catalog," Arlene G. Taylor

Distinguished Seminar Series

"Software Architecture to Support Data Translation," Sandra A. Mamrak

"Changes in the Life Cycle of Information," Toni Carbo Bearman

"Tomorrow's Library Today," W. David Penniman

"On the Nature and Function of Explanation in Intelligent Information Retrieval," Nicholas J. Belkin

"Automatic Sense Disambiguation," Michael Lesk

"Probability Theory in Information Retrieval," William S. Cooper

"Information Retrieval by Plausible Inference," W. Bruce Croft

The Research Advisory Committee

Robert M. Hayes, Dean, Graduate School of Library and Information Studies, University of California, Los Angeles

Brian Perry, Director, Research and Development Department, The British Library

Brian L. Hawkins, Vice President of Computing and Information Services, Brown University

Mervin E. Muller, Chairman and Robert M. Critchfield Professor of Engineering, Computer and Information Science Department, and Professor, Department of Statistics, The Ohio State University

Joseph H. Howard, Director, National Agricultural Library

Karen Sparck Jones, Assistant Director of Research, Computer Laboratory, University of Cambridge

Visiting Scholars

Elaine Svenonius, Professor, Graduate School of Library and Information Science, University of California, Los Angeles

Paul B. Kantor, President, Tantalus, Inc., Cleveland, Ohio

1988/89

OCLC Research Projects

"Applying Neural Networks to Classification Problems," Stuart L. Weibel

"Automated Document Architecture Processing and Tagging (ADAPT)," Stuart L. Weibel

"Bibliographic Control and Document Architecture in Hypermedia Databases," Roland Hjerppe

"Cataloger's Assistant," Diane Vizine-Goetz

"Cataloging Time and Workflow Studies," Chandra G. Prabha

"Design of Interfaces and Databases for Electronic Media (DIADEM)," Martha J. Lindeman

"Document Image Processing Toolbox," John C. Handley

"Duplicate Detection," Edward T. O'Neill

"Enhanced Bibliographic Retrieval," Martin Dillon

"The Experimental Library System (XLS)," Thomas B. Hickey

"Information Services and Scholarly Services Projects," Mark A. Crook

"Managing Large Retrievals," Chandra G. Prabha

"MARC–UP: A Prototype for Improving Retrospective Conversion," Stuart L. Weibel

"Selecting Bibliographic Record Subsets," Mark A. Crook

External and Collaborative Research

"Conversion of Academic Library Data to Machine-Readable Form," Robert E. Molyneux

"Design Principles for Third Generation Online Public Access Catalogs: Taking Account of Users and Library Use," Nicholas J. Belkin and Tefko Saracevic

"Increasing the Accessibility of the Library of Congress Subject Headings in Online Bibliographic Systems," Karen Markey Drabenstott and Diane Vizine-Goetz

"Learning Term Weights," Clement Yu

"The Library of Congress Classification in the Computer Age," Nancy J. Williamson

"The Mercury Electronic Library: A Syntactic Approach to Automatic Book Indexing," Gerard Salton

"The Use of Journals by Scholars: Implications for Designing an Interface to the Electronic Journal," Jan Olsen

Library and Information Research Grants

"Enhancing Topical Searching Using Classification Clustering," Ray R. Larson

"Knowledge-based Descriptive Cataloging of Cartographic Publications," Harold Borko and Zorana Ercegovac

"The Relationship between Library Holdings and Selection Sources," Judith Serebnick

Distinguished Seminar Series

"Parallel Computing for Information Retrieval," David L. Waltz

"A Prospectus on Information Systems Engineering," Ferdinand F. Leimkuhler

"Integrated Inquiry Systems," Karen Sparck Jones

"From Electronic Publishing to Intelligent Information Retrieval," Edward A. Fox

"Improved Access to LC Classification and LC Subject Headings for Online Searchers and Catalogers," Dagobert Soergel

"The X Window System Application Environment," David Rosenthal

Research Advisory Committee Members

Brian L. Hawkins, Vice President of Computing and Information Services, Brown University

Mervin E. Muller, Chairman and Robert M. Critchfield, Professor of Engineering, Computer and Information Science Department, The Ohio State University

Joseph H. Howard, Director, National Agricultural Library

Karen Sparck Jones, Assistant Director of Research, Computer Laboratory, University of Cambridge

Visiting Scholar

Roland Hjerppe, Group Leader, LIBLAB Library and Information Science Research Laboratory, Department of Computer and Information Science, and University Library, Linkoping University, Linkoping, Sweden

1989/90

OCLC Research Projects

"ADAPT: Automated Document Architecture Processing and Tagging," Stuart L. Weibel, John C. Handley, and Martin Dillon

"Cataloging Productivity Tools," Diane Vizine-Goetz

"Converting Machine-Readable Dewey Decimal Files," Mark A. Crook

"DIADEM: Design of Interfaces and Databases for Electronic Media," Martha J. Lindeman

"Document Image Processing Toolbox," John C. Handley

"Duplicate Detection," Edward T. O'Neill

"Enhanced Bibliographic Records," Martin Dillon

"Experimental Library System," Thomas B. Hickey

"Information and Scholarly Services," Mark A. Crook

"Information Retrieval Research Laboratory," Roger Thompson

"Interface Design Procedures," Michael J. Prasse

"The Interlibrary Loan Process," Chandra G. Prabha

"Managing Large Retrievals," Chandra G. Prabha

"Table of Contents Database," Martin Dillon

"The Video Analysis Method: Determining Usability," Michael J. Prasse

External and Collaborative Research

"Advanced Retrieval Methods for Online Catalogs," Edward A. Fox

"Back-of-the-Book Index Study," Elizabeth D. Liddy

"Balancing Local Needs with the General Good," Richard M. Dougherty and Carol Hughes

"CORE: The Chemical Online Retrieval Experiment," Lorrin Garson et al.

"Data Compression with Huffman Coding," Clement Yu and Chengwin Lui

"Improving Subject Searching in Online Catalogs," Karen Markey Drabenstott and Diane Vizine-Goetz

"Preservation," Edward T. O'Neill and Wesley L. Boomgaarden

"Using the DDC in Online Catalogs," Elizabeth E. Duncan

Library and Information Science Research Grants

"The General Structure of a Knowledge Base for Anglo-American Cataloguing Rules," Ling Hwey Jeng

"Identifying Barriers to Effective Subject Access in Library Catalogs," F.W. Lancaster

"Investigating the Structure of LCC and LCSH: Developing a Knowledge Base," Dagobert Soergel

"Toward Integration of Online Resources," Linda C. Smith

Distinguished Seminar Series

"Office of Library Programs," Anne J. Mathews

"CARL: Colorado Alliance of Research Libraries," Ward Shaw

"Demons, Paradoxes, and Golden Arches," Robert C. Heterick, Jr.

"Strategic Information Management," Donald A. Marchand

"Realistic Assessment of Information Retrieval Performance," Jeffrey Katzer

"Designing Quality User Interfaces," Robert W. Bailey

Research Advisory Committee Members

Robert C. Heterick, Jr., Vice President for Information Systems, Virginia Polytechnic and State University

Joseph H. Howard, Director, National Agricultural Library

Karen Sparck Jones, Assistant Director of Research, Computer Laboratory, University of Cambridge

Clifford A. Lynch, Director, Division of Library Automation, University of California, Oakland

1990/91

OCLC Research Projects

"ADAPT: Automated Document Architecture Processing and Tagging," Martin Dillon, John C. Handley, and Stuart L. Weibel

"Authority Control Practice in Libraries," Chandra G. Prabha

"Capturing Tables of Contents: Pilot Study," Stuart L. Weibel

"Cataloging Productivity Tools," Diane Vizine-Goetz

"Document Image Processing Toolbox," John C. Handley

"Duplicate Records in Union Catalogs," Edward T. O'Neill

"FastCat," David J. Stephens

"Information Retrieval Research Laboratory," Roger Thompson

"Interface Design Procedures," Michael J. Prasse

"Internet Resources," Martin Dillon

"Obsolete Library of Congress Subject Headings," Roy Chang

"Record Matching for Authority Control," Edward T. O'Neill

"The Usability Laboratory," Michael J. Prasse and George A. Walter

External and Collaborative Research

"Analytical Tools for Library-Generated Data," Abraham Bookstein

"Book Deterioration in Ohio Libraries," Edward T. O'Neill and Wesley L. Boomgaarden

"CORE: The Chemical Online Retrieval Experiment," Lorrin Garson et al.

"Decompression of Group 4 Image Data," Clement Yu and Chengjie Luo

Library and Information Science Research Grants

"Automatic Hierarchical Organization of Phrases Using Machine-Readable Dictionary Information," Amy J. Warner

"Determining the Content of Machine-Readable Subdivision Records," Karen Markey Drabenstott

"Expert Systems Interface to Library of Congress Subject Headings," Padmini Srinivasan

"Scholars' Access to the Documents They Cite," Keith Swigger

Distinguished Seminar Series

"Making a Science 'in' Design," John M. Carroll

"Image Databases," Howard Besser

"Information Literacy: From Hardware to Thoughtware," E. Gordon Gee

Research Advisory Committee Members

Robert C. Heterick, Jr., PhD, Vice President for Information Systems, Virginia Polytechnic and State University

Clifford A. Lynch, PhD, Director, Division of Library Automation, University of California, Oakland

Sharon J. Rogers, PhD, Assistant Vice President for Academic Affairs and University Librarian, George Washington University

Robert M. Warner, PhD, Dean of the School of Information and Library Studies, University of Michigan

1991/92

OCLC Research Projects

"Database Quality Control," Edward T. O'Neill

"Assessing Information on the Internet," Martin Dillon

"Cataloging Productivity Tools," Diane Vizine-Goetz

"Cost, Workflows, and Usage Data for Interlibrary Loan and Document Delivery," Chandra G. Prabha

"The Graphical Browse Project," Martin Dillon

"Information Retrieval Research Laboratory," Roger Thompson

"Interface Design Procedures," Michael J. Prasse

"The Selected Titles Project," David J. Stephens and Andrew Wang

External and Collaborative Research

"The Art of Back-of-the-Book Indexes," Elizabeth D. Liddy

"Book Deterioration in Ohio Libraries," Edward T. O'Neill and Wesley L. Boomgaarden

"CORE, Loren Garson," Michael Lesk, Jim Lundeen, Jan Olsen, and Stuart L. Weibel

"Design Principles for Third Generation Online Public Access Catalogs," Nicholas J. Belkin and Tefko Saracevic

"Implementation and Performance Evaluation of an Image Decompression Algorithm," Clement Yu and Chengjie Luo

Library and Information Science Research Grants

"Automatic Hierarchical Organization of Phrases Using Machine-Readable Dictionary Information," Amy J. Warner

"The Functional Components of Browsing," Barbara H. Kwasnik

"Public Libraries and the Internet/NREN," Charles R. McClure, Joe Ryan, Diana Lauterbach, and William E. Moen

"The Quality of Chinese Records in the OCLC Database," Edie Rasmussen and Marcia Lei Zeng

"Scholars' Access to the Documents They Cite," Keith Swigger

Distinguished Seminar Series

"Xanadu Worldwide Hypertext Publishing," Theodor Nelson

"User Interface Design," Ben Shneiderman

"New Technologies for Learning," Elliot Soloway

Research Advisory Committee Members

Sharon J. Rogers, PhD, Associate Vice President for Academic Affairs, George Washington University

David L. Waltz, PhD, Professor of Computer Science, Brandeis University and Director of Advanced Information Systems, Thinking Machines Corporation

Robert M. Warner, PhD, Director of the University Library, University of Michigan

Richard P. West, Associate Vice President for Information Systems and Administrative Services, University of California

Visiting Scholars

Karen M. Drabenstott, Associate Professor, School of Library and Information Studies, University of Michigan

1992/93

OCLC Research Projects

"Assessing Information on the Internet: Toward Providing Library Services for Computer-Mediated Communication," Martin Dillon and Erik Jul

"Cataloging Productivity Tools," Diane Vizine-Goetz

"Document Ranking Using Signature Files," Dik Lun Lee

"Estimating Interlibrary Loan Volume in 1993: Academic, Public, Special, and Federal Libraries," Chandra G. Prabha

"Experimental Linguistic Indexing for Information Retrieval: ELIXIR," C. Jean Godby and Bradley C. Watson

"Information Retrieval Research Laboratory," Roger Thompson and C. Jean Godby

"Modeling Users' Preferences for Document Delivery," Mark T. Kinnucan

"OCLC Authority Control," Edward T. O'Neill, W. Michael Oskins, and Kerre A. Kammerer

"Reference Client Software Design," Thomas B. Hickey

"SGML Grammar Structure," Keith E. Shafer

External and Collaborative Research

"Book Deterioration in Ohio Libraries," Edward T. O'Neill and Wesley L. Boomgaarden

"The CORE Project: Technical Shakedown and Preliminary User Studies," Stuart L. Weibel

Library and Information Science Research Grants

"Determining the Content of Machine-Readable Subdivision Records," Karen Markey Drabenstott

"Electronic Texts and Traditional Indexes: A Study of Applicability and Performance," Elizabeth D. Liddy

"Measuring Diversity in Public Library Collections," Judith Serenick and Frank Quinn

Distinguished Seminar Series

"Rushing Toward 2000: Enhancing Services, Technologies, and Priorities for Resource Sharing," Mary E. Jackson

"Economics of Scholarly Publishing," Roger G. Noll

"Toward a National Collaboratory," Daniel E. Atkins

"Foundations for Automatic Summarizing," Karen Sparck Jones

Research Advisory Committee Members

David L. Waltz, PhD, Vice President of the Computer Science Research Division, NEC Research Institute

Richard P. West, Associate Vice President for Information Systems and Administrative Services, University of California

Look Costers, Director of the Centre for Library Automation Pica, the Netherlands

Edward Emil David, Jr., ScD, Industrial Consultant with a research specialty of electrical engineering and former President, Exxon Research and Engineering Company

Visiting Scholars

Mark T. Kinnucan, Associate Professor, School of Library and Information Science, University of Western Ontario

Dik L. Lee, Associate Professor, Computer and Information Science, The Ohio State University

1993/94

OCLC Research Projects

"Integrating Guidon with the World Wide Web," Thomas B. Hickey

"Cuttering for the Library of Congress Classification," Edward T. O'Neill

"Manifestations of Fiction Works," Edward T. O'Neill

"Cataloging Productivity Tools," Diane Vizine-Goetz

"Scholarly Publishing on the World Wide Web," Stuart L. Weibel

"The LC-OCLC CIP Project," Chandra G. Prabha

"Manipulating Tagged Text," Keith E. Shafer

"Translating Mathematical Markup for Electronic Journals," Keith E. Shafer

"Two Techniques for the Identification of Phrases in Full Text," C. Jean Godby

"Converting ACM Authors' Articles to SGML," Bradley C. Watson

"Evolving Issues and Trends in Interlibrary Loan and Document Delivery," Chandra G. Prabha

External and Collaborative Research

"OCLC's Participation in the TULIP Project," Thomas B. Hickey

"The Design and Implementation of XSCEPTER, and X-Windows Graphical Users Interface to the CORE Project," Stuart L. Weibel

"A Study of Libraries Using the Dewey Decimal Classification in the OCLC Online Union Catalog," Joan S. Mitchell and Mark A. Crook

"A System for Analyzing Cataloging Rules," Shoichi Taniguchi

Library and Information Science Research Grants

"Enhancing a New Design for Subject Access to Online Catalogs," Karen M. Drabenstott

"An Empirical Test of Gopher Searching Using Three Organization Schemes," C. Olivia Frost and Joseph Janes

"Toward the Bibliographic Control of Works," Richard P. Smiraglia and Gregory H. Leazer

"Evaluating Public Library Fiction Collections," James J. Sweetland and Judith J. Senkevitch

Distinguished Seminar Series

"One Journal Editor's View of the Future of Journals," Donald H. Kraft

"SGML to Braille, Large Print, and Audio," Yuri Rubinsky

Research Advisory Committee Members

David L. Waltz, PhD, Vice President of the Computer Science Research Division, NEC Research Institute

Richard P. West, Associate Vice President for Information Systems and Administrative Services, University of California

Look Costers, Director of the Centre for Library Automation Pica, the Netherlands

Edward Emil David, Jr., ScD, Industrial Consultant with a research specialty of electrical engineering and former President, Exxon Research and Engineering Company

Clifford A. Lynch, PhD, Director, Division of Library Automation, University of California, Oakland

Carol A. Mandel, MSLS, MA, Deputy University Librarian, Columbia University

Visiting Scholars

Shoichi Taniguchi, Research Associate, University of Library and Information Science, Ibaraki-ken, Japan

1994/95

OCLC Research Projects

"Business-oriented Research and Planning," Mark A. Crook

"Adding Holdings Information to CIP Records before Book Receipt," Chandra G. Prabha

"Characteristics of Publications Sought through OCLC PRISM Interlibrary Loan," Chandra G. Prabha

"Copy Cataloging Practices: Use of the Call Number by Dewey Libraries," Edward T. O'Neill and Patrick McClain

"Dewey 2000," Diane Vizine-Goetz and Joan S. Mitchell

"World Wide Web Access to Fred," Jonathan R. Fausey and Keith E. Shafer

"Guidon Web: Applying Java to Scholarly Electronic Journals," Thomas B. Hickey

"The PURL Project," Keith E. Shafer, Stuart L. Weibel, and Erik Jul

"Embedded Systems Experience and Views," Roger Thompson and Keith E. Shafer

"Arbitrary SGML Viewers and Their Role in Online Text Delivery Systems," Bradley C. Watson

"STORD–Structured Text on Relational Databases," Thomas B. Hickey and Thomas L. Terrall

"Using SiteSearch to Create a Resource Discovery Tool for the Internet," C. Jean Godby

"Issues of Document Description in HTML," Eric J. Miller

External and Collaborative Research

"Feasibility of a Computer-generated Subject Validation File Based on Frequency of Occurrence of Assigned LC Subject Headings," Lois Mai Chan and Diane Vizine-Goetz

"Metadata: The Foundation of Resource Description," Stuart L. Weibel

Library and Information Science Research Grants

"The Effect of Linkage Structure on Retrieval Performance and User Response in a Hypertext-based Bibliographic Retrieval System," Alexandra Dimitroff and Dietmar Wolfram

"Developing Control Mechanisms for Intellectual Access for Discipline-based Virtual Libraries: A Study of the Process," Marcia Lei Zeng

Distinguished Seminar Series

"Electronic Reference in Academic Libraries in the 1990s," Carol Tenopir

Research Advisory Committee Members

Edward Emil David, Jr., ScD, Industrial Consultant with a research specialty of electrical engineering and former President, Exxon Research and Engineering Company

Clifford A. Lynch, PhD, Director, Division of Library Automation, University of California, Oakland

Carol A. Mandel, MSLS, MA, Deputy University Librarian, Columbia University

Joseph Hardin, BA, Associate Director, Software Development Group, National Center for Supercomputing Applications, University of Illinois, Urbana-Champaign

1995/96

OCLC Research Projects

"Four-Figure Cutter Tables," Edward T. O'Neill, Brian F. Lavoie, Jeffrey A. Young, and Patrick D. McClain

"Automatic Subject Assignment via the Scorpion System," Keith E. Shafer

"Characteristics of Articles Requested through Interlibrary Loan," Chandra G. Prabha

"Characteristics of Book Collections in Academic Research Libraries," Chandra G. Prabha

"Classification Research at OCLC," Diane Vizine-Goetz

"Enhancing the Indexing Vocabulary of the Dewey Decimal Classification," C. Jean Godby

"Evaluating a Multiprocessor NT Server for Z39.50 Use," Thomas B. Hickey, Richard Bennett, and Thomas L. Terrall

"FirstSearch Next Generation: Another Look at FirstSearch," Thomas B. Hickey, Jenny Colvard, and Thomas L. Terrall

"Image Description on the Internet: Summary of CNI/OCLC Image Metadata Workshop," Stuart L. Weibel and Eric J. Miller

"Kilroy: An Internet Research Project," Keith E. Shafer

"A Metalanguage for Describing Internet Resources," C. Jean Godby and Eric Miller

"Mr. Dui's Topic Finder," Mark W. Bendig

"Use of the PURL Service," Keith E. Shafer

"Visualizing Spatial Relationships between Internet Objects," Eric J. Miller

External and Collaborative Research

"The Bosnian National Library: Building a Virtual Collection," Edward T. O'Neill, Jeffrey A. Young, and Robert Bremer

"Feasibility of a Computer-Generated Subject Validation File Based on Frequency of Occurrence of Assigned Subject Headings: Phase II, Nature and Patterns of Invalid Headings," Lois Mai Chan and Diane Vizine-Goetz

"The Monticello Project: Design Considerations for a Virtual Library," Eric J. Miller, Tod Matola, Pat Stevens, and Jay Hayden

"The Warwick Metadata Workshop: A Framework for the Deployment of Resource Description," Lorcan Dempsey and Stuart L. Weibel

Library and Information Science Research Grants

"Analyzing the Viability of Using Peer Group Holdings as an Evaluation Tool for Public Library Adult Fiction," James H. Sweetland and Judith J. Senkevitch

"An Experimental Study on Graphical Tables of Contents," Xia Lin

"The Impact of Electronic Journals on Scholarly Communication: A Reference and Citation Study," Stephen P. Harter

"A Relational Thesaurus: Modeling Semantic Relationships Using Frames," Rebecca Green

Distinguished Seminar Series

"Cataloging Rules and Conceptual Models," Barbara B. Tillet

"The Copyright Dilemma: Legal Tensions and Information Networks," Kenneth Crews

Research Advisory Committee Members

Edward Emil David, Jr., ScD, Industrial Consultant with a research specialty of electrical engineering and former President, Exxon Research and Engineering Company

Clifford A. Lynch, PhD, Director, Division of Library Automation, University of California, Oakland

Carol A. Mandel, MSLS, MA, Deputy University Librarian, Columbia University

Joseph Hardin, BA, Associate Director, Software Development Group, National Center for Supercomputing Applications, University of Illinois, Urbana-Champaign

Visiting Scholars

John V. Richardson, Jr., Associate Professor, Graduate School of Education and Information Studies, University of California at Los Angeles

New Electronic Scholarship and Libraries; Or the Medium Became the Message

Sharon J. Rogers
Charlene S. Hurt

Nine years ago a radically different world of scholarly communication was proposed on the back page of the *Chronicle of Higher Education*[1] suggesting a way to transform scholarly communication through the medium of electronic publishing. By implication, the article predicted the end of scholarly journals in the form they currently existed. They would be replaced by a networked scholarly communication system developed and controlled by institutions of higher education and scholarly associations. The hypothesized system encompassed all elements of scholarly production: preprints, informal intellectual comment and exchange, peer reviewing, citation monitoring, formal publication, indexing and abstracting, and archiving. The system sought to combine the strengths of on-line publishing (speed, wide distribution, interactivity) with the strengths of traditional scholarly publishing (blind peer reviews, selectivity, indexing and archiving). The new system envisioned would assist libraries in meeting the soaring costs of journal subscriptions, the constant demand for additional space, and the high cost of maintaining paper journal collections. An important aspect of the proposal was the role of universities, which, by gaining control of the scholarly publication process, would also gain control over the mechanism that dominates the faculty reward system.

Sharon J. Rogers is a Library Consultant, Arlington, VA.

Charlene S. Hurt is University Librarian, Georgia State University, Atlanta, GA.

[Haworth co-indexing entry note]: "New Electronic Scholarship and Libraries; Or the Medium Became the Message." Rogers, Sharon J, and Charlene S. Hurt. Co-published simultaneously in *Journal of Library Administration* (The Haworth Press, Inc.) Vol. 25, No. 4, 1998, pp. 239-249; and: *OCLC 1967-1997: Thirty Years of Furthering Access to the World's Information* (ed: K. Wayne Smith) The Haworth Press, Inc., 1998, pp. 239-249. Single or multiple copies of this article are available for a fee from The Haworth Document Delivery Service [1-800-342-9678, 9:00 a.m. - 5:00 p.m. (EST). E-mail address: getinfo@haworthpressinc.com].

More explicitly, the 1989 article suggested that

> the new scholarly communication system would provide many benefits to colleges and universities, including substantial economic advantages:

- The amount of money spent by colleges and universities on subscriptions to publications would be substantially reduced and the savings used for the new system. In just ten years, the average costs of research journals have increased 160 percent, and it is likely that trend will continue. And more than 5,000 new journals, some in new fields, began publication in 1988 alone–creating even more pressure on already ailing library budgets.
- The need for more library space would be reduced. The escalation in size and number of journals creates a constant need for more space to house the publications and their readers. In 1989, each square foot of new library space costs an average of $95.43.
- The hours spent processing journals, shelving, and reshelving them could be much better spent on developing more sophisticated indexes of journal contents and on helping users find and select the information they want.

> As a bonus, the system would establish and enforce standards for the formats used for storing data, thus assuring scholars that materials computerized now will be easily retrievable in the future.

> Most important, however, universities would regain control over decisions made about the largest item in their budgets: faculty salaries. Instead of letting publishers and an inner circle of referees decide who gets published and, therefore, who receives tenure and merit raises, universities could insure the quality and fairness of the review of research in all fields. Universities would have a prescribed role in choosing the members of review and management boards. The reviewers chosen by such boards could be very different from the people now used by journals if the selections were not based on the buddy system or "old boy" connections. The system thus could provide better information for universities to make informed personnel judgements.

> If universities, foundations, libraries, and scholarly organizations act now to form this new communication system, it could soon be in place to serve the needs of researchers and scholars far into the 21st century.[2]

The reactions to the article were fairly equally divided between praise and indignation, with one group of scholarly publishers inviting the authors to attend their annual meeting to "defend" their ideas, and other readers wanting to know how they could contribute to beginning the revolution. It was apparent that there were a significant number of vested interests that would have to be considered in any proposed solution, and that the obstacles to the vision were primarily organizational, personal and cultural. Only by overcoming entrenched positions of the various stake-holders could the benefits be realized.

The higher education community was not sufficiently organized to enable such an inclusive approach, however. In the intervening years, a series of separate initiatives developed, undertaken by the various stake-holders. The most comprehensive initiative was announced late in 1995 by the Association of American Universities (AAU) and the Association of Research Libraries (ARL). The goal was to distribute scholarly work online to facilitate scholarly publishing based on the cost of information, rather than "cost-plus."[3] If the plan had been realized, all 58 members of the AAU would have contributed $30,000 each to create a $1.7 million fund to create a not-for-profit entity. The proposal was silent on the crucial issue of peer review, an essential element to maintain the trust and confidence of the academic community in the quality of the work that was being distributed.

Despite the lack of central direction, however, electronic publishing of scholarly journals grew at impressive rates during the last several years. The sixth edition of the Association for Research Libraries' *Directory of Electronic Journals, Newsletters and Academic Discussion Lists*[4] includes 1,093 journal titles, 596 newsletters and 3,188 discussion lists. Of these three categories, electronic journals increased the most: 257 percent over last year's total of 306. There is also an increase in the number of titles for which a fee is charged: up to 168 titles, or 11 percent of the total. In 1994, only 29 titles were available on a fee basis. There is an even greater increase in titles using peer review: 600 percent more than in 1994 to 517 titles.

OCLC recognized early that the times were right to create a new way to meet its public mission of furthering access to information and reducing information costs by creating options for libraries within the electronic publishing environment. Its achievements were perhaps best summarized in a 1996 news release from the American Institute of Physics which stated, "AIP and the remainder of the scientific and technical publishing community owe an enormous debt of gratitude to OCLC for its ground-breaking efforts in online journal publishing. OCLC made a high-risk, multimillion-dollar investment in the development of its EJO system and Guidon client, at a time when the World Wide Web was yet to be invented. Clearly their efforts have advanced the development of online journals at a much faster pace than would otherwise have been the case."[5]

OCLC claimed the demonstration of electronic publishing capability as its contribution to realizing the vision of a revolutionized system of scholarly communication. In a 1994 *OCLC Newsletter* article, it identified the technical requirements for success in an electronic publishing venture:

- electronic journals must provide all of the information found in print journals, including color and black-and-white images, equations and tables
- electronic versions must go beyond the print to take full advantage of the electronic medium: faster publication of important information, decoupled from the constraints of publishing "by the issue," as well as printing and mailing delays; comprehensive searching and browsing of the entire journal, rather than just an issue; ease of use and access from offices, dorms and homes 24 hours a day; access through a single interface to related and relevant information of all kinds, including bibliographic references and reactions to the journal articles from other researchers.[6]

Beginning in the mid-1980s, OCLC developed the Electronic Information Delivery Online System (EIDOS) which conceptualized an electronic book with searchable table of contents and index pages combined with actual text and graphics. The prototype envisioned a split screen with simultaneous views of index and text. Recognizing the coming power of networking, OCLC anticipated storing the text and images centrally, while storing the tables of contents and indexing locally. Another OCLC research project was Graph-Text which could produce the typographic equivalent of a fully searchable text as it appeared in its original publication. Zoom features would allow a user to enlarge specific areas of a page to examine details and individual pages could be printed at the desktop. A compact disc was perceived as the medium of delivery.

By 1991, the demonstrations had moved into a production model that was used to launch an online, peer-reviewed journal in partnership with the American Association for the Advancement of Science (AAAS), the *Online Journal of Current Clinical Trials* (OJCCT). It was the first electronic journal to support graphs, tables and illustrations as well as mathematical equations. It was the first to provide typeset-quality text through an interface called Guidon. The Guidon interface was based on software called Newton which was developed for the OCLC EPIC service, an OCLC online reference system. At the same time, it used OCLC's investment in EPIC and the OCLC FirstSearch service to provide hypertext links to MEDLINE, the citation database of the National Library of Medicine, and its abstracts. By the time of release 3.0 in December 1994, Guidon provided color and gray-scale graphics, a link to FirstSearch, a "new since last logon" feature, a current feature, boxed information in sidebars, email to the publisher, email requests for information to advertisers, and the capability to produce backfiles on CD-ROM.

Even more important, OJCCT realized the element of the 1989 visionary model by giving physicians faster access to research results on new and re-examined medical treatments. It eliminated the month or more spent preparing an accepted article for publication and by-passed the delays and vagaries of the mail system. This achievement could only be realized because OJCCT became the first electronic journal to be indexed in *Index Medicus* and its MEDLINE database. The struggle for success with OJCCT was not with the concept, which was an adaptation of the conventional peer-review model of scholarly publishing. It was not with the technology which OCLC had developed. The struggle was with the risk-taking behavior of faculty and researchers to publish in a new medium, not trusting its ultimate acceptance as a scholarly communication tool. Under the AAAS/OCLC partnership, 30 articles were published. The journal is now owned by Chapman & Hall.

But the breakthrough had been made. Patricia A. Morgan, Director of publications for the AAAS, declared, "As far as I'm concerned, we now have a template for electronic, scholarly publishing. And this template is solid. It's been tested like very few projects have been tested."[7] And, by 1995, the Electronic Journals Online (EJO) program had added several journals to *Current Clinical Trials: The Online Journal of Knowledge Synthesis for Nursing,* published by Sigma Theta Tau International Honor Society of Nursing; *Electronic Letters Online,* published by the Institution of Electrical Engineers; *Applied Physics Letters Online* from the American Institute of Physics; *Immunology Today Online,* from Elsevier Science Publishers; and two clusters of journals from Current Science (*Current Opinions in Biology* with 6 journals and *Current Opinions in Medicine* with 24 journals).

Then the comet of the World Wide Web swept across the sky of electronic publishing, making proprietary interfaces, such as Guidon, obsolete almost overnight. The World Wide Web also made individuals and groups into instant publishers and the landscape of scholarly publishing fragmented with the joys of entrepreneurial experimentation. Almost daily new initiatives, large and small, were springing up to tantalize with their possibilities. Each of the electronic scholarly publishing initiatives has its unique set of characteristics, with varying strengths and weaknesses. Some representative examples follow.

Project MUSE

Project MUSE, begun in 1995, is an initiative of the Johns Hopkins University Press and the Milton S. Eisenhower Library (Johns Hopkins). Currently funded by the National Endowment for the Humanities and The Andrew W. Mellon Foundation, Project MUSE provides networked access to the full text of the Press' 40 scholarly journals. Marketed to libraries, Project MUSE allows access to the entire campus, with no limits on simultaneous users. Faculty, students and staff of a subscribing institution may distribute articles freely within the contiguous campus community, allowing users to download, print and make unlimited paper copies for classroom or personal use. Libraries may store archival copies in a variety of mediums, including paper, CD-ROM and microfilm. Project MUSE focuses on current issues, with some backfiles as far back as 1994. New issues are placed online in advance of paper distribution. The online journals include all graphics and text.

JSTOR

JSTOR was originally conceived by William G. Bowen, President of The Andrew W. Mellon Foundation, which sponsored a pilot project to test the concept. JSTOR is now an independent nonprofit organization, which was provided with its initial working capital by the Mellon Foundation and is now expected to become self-sustaining. The basic idea of JSTOR is to convert the back issues of paper journals into electronic formats, to achieve savings in space while simultaneously improving access to the journal content. It was also viewed as a solution to preservation problems. The project began with the backfiles of ten journals in economics and history, from volume I, number 1 to 1990, and is planned to expand to 100 important scholarly journals in a variety of fields. The bit-mapped images of each page are linked to a text file generated with optical character recognition (OCR) software which, along with newly constructed Table-of-Contents indexes, permits complete search and retrieval of the journal material.

Academic Press' IDEAL

IDEAL is a project of Academic Press, which mounts the complete text of 175 Academic Press journals, from 1996 to the present (plus some 1995 issues). Anyone with Internet access can browse and search tables of contents and abstracts; authorized users can view, search, print and download complete articles in the Acrobat format. IDEAL offers a site license aimed at large consortia which provides access to all sites within a licensed consortium to all the journals formerly held in print form anywhere within the consortium (if the consortium is large enough, this is all 175 titles). This permits copying and transmitting of articles within the consortium, plus unlimited use for course packs, but prohibits all copying and transmitting of the electronic files outside the consortium. Other publishers are being invited to make their journals available on IDEAL. This project does not appear to have grant support, and seems designed to guarantee Academic Press a constant flow of income by charging consortia a percentage of their paper subscription costs provided they do not cancel paper subscriptions.

Springer-Verlag's LINK Information Service

In 1997, Springer-Verlag announced the LINK information service, which intends to provide all 400 journals of the international publishing group, as well as electronic books. About 150 titles are currently available. Generally, LINK information service users have access to the electronic version before the printed counterpart. As in IDEAL, table of contents and abstracts can be read by all; LINK also provides for full-text search. Only subscribers can access complete articles. It appears that LINK will be marketed in similar ways to IDEAL, with protection of their revenue from print services, but limited information is currently available.

By July 1997, Mignon Adams recognized that all of this experimentation was developing into five emerging models for scientific journals online: table-of-contents/document delivery; single journals on the Web; publishers' collections on the Web; index/abstract with links to full text; and search engines for library subscriptions.[8] She concludes that "earlier dreams of researchers' taking back the dissemination of their findings will probably not be realized. Instead, commercial publishers are creating models that will maintain costs at previous levels."[9]

OCLC's 1997 development of the OCLC FirstSearch Electronic Collections Online service (ECO) is demonstration of the last model sited above, as well as the culmination of more than a decade of OCLC research and development. A major breakthrough is that publishers have granted OCLC archival rights to journals in the collection. John Barnes, director of OCLC Electronic Journals Division, described the service as giving "libraries the quality and perpetual access they have always received with print subscriptions coupled with the added searching power and space savings of electronic documents."[10] To view abstracts and articles, the library must subscribe to journals, either directly with publishers or through publisher subscription agents. OCLC maintains the complete profile of the journals in the collections, along with the subscription start and end dates and links it to the library's access account. The library's rights to the archive remain active regardless of current subscription status. By early 1998, the service is expected to provide access to more than 500 journals from 16 publishers. Also in 1998, ECO will be integrated with the FirstSearch service (OCLC's menu-driven end-user system that provides access to more than 60 databases of bibliographic, abstract and full-text information, introduced in 1991) in order to provide seamless access to bibliographic databases and online full text through a single interface. With this link in place, FirstSearch users will be able to search and browse within their Electronic Collections Online collection, or access journal articles from links to abstracting and indexing and bibliographic databases.[11] FirstSearch enables the 1989 vision of the authors by making the article, rather than the journal, a widely available unit of scholarly communication.

Given this impressive growth in the number and variety of electronic scholarly journals, is the 1989 scholarly communication system emerging? The answer is that the medium has become the message. The medium of electronic and technical capacity the authors anticipated would transform scholarly publishing has prevailed. The message of taking control of the scholarly output of institutions of higher education and using the electronic and technical capabilities to dramatically change scholarly *communication* has been lost.

It is easy to recognize some of the factors that contribute to this outcome. The joyful exuberance of experimentation has been noted above. The profit motive of many stakeholders looms large, from the very large and increasingly consolidated publishers of scholarly journals to the professional associations that depend on the income from their professional journals. With the increasingly large conglomerates controlling scholarly publishing, higher education may be in greater danger than ever of losing control over the elements of scholarly communication, which force them to pay three and four times over for the same publication effort. The urge to protect or stake out turf prevails in both the experimental and established publishing arenas, preventing collaborations that would appear to save both money and effort. It is probably impossible to get an accurate count of the number of "national digital library" projects that have been announced. Finally, the failure to deal with the gatekeeping role of editors of scholarly publications and to provide a systematic model for peer review ensures that the basic conservatism of the academy will triumph.

The basic conservatism of the academy was recognized in the *Online Journal of Current Clinical Trials* context in 1994 when "a new journal in an unorthodox format that could be read only on a computer screen was not thought to be the place to publish papers that might lead to tenure, promotion, better salaries, and more grant money."[12] Little in this culture has changed. In a recent announcement, editors of the American Psychological Association journals advised APA members "not to post draft, accepted, or published papers on the Internet or World Wide Web, because such papers will not be accepted by most of the APA journals, the *New England Journal of Medicine,* or *Neuroscience.*"[13] The *Chronicle of Higher Education* recently reported that some students at Virginia Polytechnic Institute and State University have refused to publish their dissertations on-line, for fear that would interfere with getting the research published later.[14]

But the urge to attempt to change the culture is apparent. In August 1997, Columbia University Press unveiled Columbia International Affairs Online (CIAO), developed over three years with support from the Mellon Foundation. CIAO is an on-line service of papers-in-progress combined with abstracts from selected journals, conference schedules and full texts of selected books published by Columbia. At the same time, The American Political Science Association is attempting to replace the "paper room" service of professional association meetings by providing about 150 papers from its recent annual meeting on a web site jointly run by Harvard University's library.[15]

In 1991, when K. Wayne Smith, President and CEO of OCLC, participated in launching the *Online Journal of Current Clinical Trials,* he noted that the revolution was not just in journal publishing, but in "journal reading. There are hypertext links within the document and external links to other databases, which means that you can consult with other sources at the same time, on the same system. You can profile the information according to your needs."[16] This radical change in the way reading occurs is not uniformly seen as desirable. In an August 15, 1997, "Point of View" in *The Chronicle of Higher Education,*" David Rothenberg reflects on "How the Web Destroys the Quality of Students' Research Papers," noting that "the placelessness of the Web leads to an ethereal randomness of thought. Gone are the pathways of logic and passion, the sense of the progress of an argument. Chance holds sway, and it more often misses than hits."[17] The same concern is reflected in a provocative article titled "Revolution in the Library," by Gertrude Himmelfarb, who says, "The medium itself is too fluid, too mobile and volatile, to encourage any sustained effort of thought."[18] This discomfort with electronic publishing is in large part a product of the turbulence of the current electronic environment, which many see as a temporary condition. The efforts of organizations like OCLC to retain the traditional strengths of scholarly publishing while enhancing the accessibility of information are essential to overcoming these fears. So is greater affordability of multimedia technology and archiving, which can add value to electronic publications in ways barely hinted at so far.

Himmelfarb demonstrates the depth of the transition required by providing historical prospective, describing the print revolution as a "perfect example of the principle of quantity transmuted into quality. The quantum leap in the number of books now available to each individual or library is almost the least of the consequences of that revolution. More significant is its democratizing effect–the liberation of the culture from the control of clerics and scribes."[19] She goes on to discuss the electronic revolution as an attempt to take that democratizing process a step forward, in that the reader is "not only the recipient of all this information but the creator of it, an active partner in this 'interactive process.' "[20]

In summary, the electronic revolution in journal publishing so far has only resulted in a quantum leap in the number of journals available. The democratizing effect envisioned in 1989 with a new scholarly communication system has not been realized. A number of factors contribute to this, including a lack of faith in the stability of the network, lack of confidence in technology, a general discomfort with online research and a high cost of multimedia publication. The scholarly community, including its institutions of higher education and professional associations, failed to seize the opportunity to take control of their scholarly output, and publishers have been unable to develop satisfactory economic models for electronic publishing that fully exploit the potential of the new medium. Efforts such as those at OCLC, Project MUSE and JSTOR show what can be done. For electronic publishing to prevail, however, it must move beyond merely reproducing print. Perhaps the 21st century will heed the words of Aldous Huxley:

It has become obvious that the machine is here to stay . . . The sensible thing to do is not to revolt against the inevitable, but to use and modify it, to make it serve your purposes. Machines exist; let us then exploit them to create beauty–a modern beauty, while we are about it.[21]

NOTES

1. Rogers, Sharon J. and Charlene S. Hurt. 1989. "How Scholarly Communication Should Work in the 21st Century." *The Chronicle of Higher Education* (October 18): A56.

2. Rogers and Hurt. Ibid.

3. Jacobson, Robert L. 1995. "Research Universities Consider Plan to Distribute Scholarly Work Online." *The Chronicle of Higher Education* (November 3): A32.

4. *ARL: a Bimonthly Newsletter of Research Library Issues and Actions.* 1996. Washington, DC: Association for Research Libraries. Issue 187 (August).

5. American Institute of Physics. 1996. "Applied Physics Letters Online moves from OCLC to AIP." Press Release, December 2.

6. Keyhani, Andrea. 1994. "OCLC electronic publishing: creating new pathways to information." *OCLC Newsletter* (September/October) No. 211: 15-17.

7. Wilson, David L. 1994. "A Journal's Big Break; National Library of Medicine will index an electronic journal on MEDLINE." *The Chronicle of Higher Education* (January 26): A23, A25.

8. Adams, Mignon. 1997. "Scientific Journals Online: Five Emerging Models," Library Issues: briefings for faculty and administrators Vol. 17, No. 6 (July).

9. Adams: 4.

10. Barnes, John. 1997. "Electronic Collections Online is here," *OCLC Newsletter* (July/August) No. 228: 24.

11. Nilges, Chip. 1997. "Integration is key feature." *OCLC Newsletter* (July/August) No. 228: 26.

12. Wilson: A23.

13. "Internet Publication Warning." 1997. *Change* (May/June): 9.

14. "Virginia Tech Graduate Students Balk at On-Line Dissertations." 1997. *The Chronicle of Higher Education* (May 9): A28.

15. "Hot Type." 1997. *The Chronicle of Higher Education* (September 5): A26.

16. Smith, K. Wayne. 1991. Remarks, Press Conference, American Association for the Advancement of Science, Washington, DC, September 24.

17. Rothenberg, David. 1997. "How the Web Destroys the Quality of Students' Research Papers." *The Chronicle of Higher Education* (August 15): A44.

18. Himmelfarb, Gertrude. 1997. "Revolution in the Library." *American Scholar* Spring 1997, reprinted in *The Key Reporter.* Vol. 62 No. 3 (spring): 1-5.

19. Himmelfarb: 2.

20. Himmelfarb: 2.

21. quoted in Rawlins, Gregory J. E. 1992. "The New Publishing: Technology's Impact on the Publishing Industry Over the Next Decade," *The Public Access Computer Systems Review* 3, No. 8: 42.

OCLC:
Yesterday, Today and Tomorrow

K. Wayne Smith

OCLC: YESTERDAY

The technological history of OCLC is well known: the introduction of online shared cataloging in 1971 and the resulting dramatic savings for libraries in cataloging costs; the expansion of the OCLC network over the past 26 years from 54 Ohio libraries to 25,000 libraries in 63 countries; the sustained growth of the OCLC shared bibliographic database, WorldCat, to its present status as the most consulted database in higher education; and the recent pioneering work in end-user online reference services, electronic publishing and electronic archiving.

Appendix A provides an overview of the products, services and technological platforms that OCLC has introduced (and discontinued) since 1971. In its first decade, OCLC focused its efforts on creating and expanding the online cataloging system and the telecommunications network and adding subsystems to complete the design of the original system. In the 1980s, OCLC began adapting distributed computing and microcomputing technologies as its product and service line expanded to some 60 offerings. The organization also began to look at ways it could "move beyond bibliography" by furnishing information not only to library staffs, but to library patrons. In the 1990s, OCLC put in place a new telecommunications network and a new online system for cataloging and resource sharing. OCLC also launched a major, new core business in reference services.

K. Wayne Smith is President and Chief Executive Officer, OCLC Online Computer Library Center, Inc.

[Haworth co-indexing entry note]: "OCLC: Yesterday, Today and Tomorrow." Smith, K. Wayne. Co-published simultaneously in *Journal of Library Administration* (The Haworth Press, Inc.) Vol. 25, No. 4, 1998, pp. 251-270; and: *OCLC 1967-1997: Thirty Years of Furthering Access to the World's Information* (ed: K. Wayne Smith) The Haworth Press, Inc., 1998, pp. 251-270. Single or multiple copies of this article are available for a fee from The Haworth Document Delivery Service [1-800-342-9678, 9:00 a.m. - 5:00 p.m. (EST). E-mail address: getinfo@haworthpressinc.com].

In short, over three decades, OCLC has moved steadily toward fulfilling its vision–to provide information to people when and where they need it, in the form they want, and at a price they can afford.

Technology, however, is only part of the OCLC story. Less chronicled, but equally important, is the evolution of OCLC as an organization. The author submits that OCLC's nonprofit status, financial philosophy, and membership role in governance have provided a unique and necessary framework for the organization to successfully adapt and evolve through 30 years of continuous technological change.

Nonprofit Status

OCLC was founded as a nonprofit corporation in 1967 by Frederick G. Kilgour and the Ohio College Association, a group consisting of the presidents of Ohio's 54 private and public colleges and universities. OCLC was one of the first institutions designed specifically to help colleges and universities cope with the information explosion, not only through using new technology, but through using old-fashioned library cooperation and resource sharing.

Peter Dobkin Hall identifies nonprofit organizations as bodies of individuals who associate for any of three major purposes: (1) to perform public tasks that have been delegated to them by the state; (2) to perform public tasks for which there is a demand that neither the state nor for-profit organizations are willing to fulfill; and (3) to influence the direction of policy in the state, the for-profit sector, or other nonprofit organizations.[1]

The newly-created OCLC was basically of the second category. None of the academic institutions could do singly what they intended to do cooperatively through OCLC. At that time, the for-profit sector had no apparent interest in operating a library network. And in the government sector, the Library of Congress, already overwhelmed with existing priorities, was reluctant to take on another large, resource-consuming commitment.

From the reports and writings of those involved in the founding of OCLC, it is clear that they never contemplated establishing OCLC as a commercial enterprise or as a traditional vendor of services. From the start, the founders envisioned OCLC as a nonprofit institution dedicated to furthering scholarship and education. OCLC's objectives were not to maximize profits or return on shareholders' investment, but to increase availability of library resources among Ohio's academic libraries and to reduce the rate of rise of per-unit library costs. Its broad public purpose mission was to "further access to the ever-expanding body of worldwide scientific, educational and literary knowledge and information."

OCLC's founders were men and women of academe. They brought to OCLC not only the ideals of research, scholarship, teaching and outreach associated with their academic backgrounds, but also the ideals of librarianship, particularly American librarianship's holy grail—the democratization of access to information.

Moreover, the founder-in-chief, Frederick G. Kilgour, had worked as a librarian and a library director at Harvard and Yale for nearly a quarter of a century. He had also lectured on the history of science and medicine at Yale. He brought to OCLC a rare combination of skills—a lifelong student and scholar, an historian who looks to the future, an entrepreneur who knows how to manage, and a dreamer who knows how to get things done. If, as Emerson has said, an institution is the lengthened shadow of a person, then for OCLC, that person is Fred Kilgour.

From the outset, research, scholarship, teaching and outreach were part of OCLC's core corporate values. In the ensuing years, because of its nonprofit status, OCLC would be regularly called upon by the library community to subsidize good works such as the CONSER (Conversion of Serials) Program and the U.S. Newspaper Program—programs that could not have been accomplished without an institution such as OCLC.

Financial Philosophy

A second defining characteristic of OCLC has been its financial independence. Although OCLC is a nonprofit organization, its financial performance has always been taken seriously and treated as a priority. From the beginning, the founders were determined that OCLC should pay its own way. Each of its three presidents has clearly understood that OCLC cannot do any public good if it is broke. Thus, OCLC's financial policy, according to the first annual report, called "for each institution to pay for operational costs prorated on the amount of use each member makes of the system."[2]

That statement was echoed 25 years later in the 1991/92 OCLC Annual Report:

> While a nonprofit corporation, OCLC has always held the belief that it must maintain a strong financial base from which to pursue its broad public purposes. Accordingly, OCLC funds its operations and its research and development with revenues generated by services provided to participating libraries and does not rely on government appropriations, foundation funding, or membership assessments.[3]

It is also worth noting that OCLC's public purposes of furthering access to the world's information and reducing information costs have always dominated its plans and programs. Throughout OCLC's history, on any significant matter involving prices and charges to the membership, there has always been full disclosure, lengthy due process, and open communications between OCLC, its U.S. regional networks and member libraries.

In essence, OCLC is both a nonprofit organization and a business and it must be good at being both. Each of its presidents has worked hard to maintain a strong financial base. OCLC has always been and remains totally self-supporting. In 30 years of operations, OCLC has never charged its members an assessment or had a deficit year. In 30 years of operations, OCLC has had only $50,000 in bad debt. Revenues, which totaled some $155 million in fiscal 1997, come entirely from user fees. OCLC's financial track record has enabled it, when necessary, to borrow money in the form of industrial revenue bonds. Over the years, OCLC has borrowed nearly $110 million in such bonds issued by Franklin County, Ohio, and purchased by institutional and individual investors throughout the country. This is the best evidence the author can offer of the confidence the general financial community has in the way OCLC has been managed.

By always operating in a prudent and businesslike manner, OCLC has been able to accommodate growth, replace and modernize facilities, conduct necessary research and development, and still subsidize worthwhile projects for the benefit of the library community. For example, during the author's eight-year tenure alone, OCLC has returned over $45 million in credits, price cuts, and subsidies to member libraries. In 1996 and 1997, OCLC subsidized the purchase of some 5,000 new, state-of-the-art workstations for its members so they can participate more fully in the World Wide Web. And, over the past thirty years, OCLC's prices have consistently been one of the best bargains in the library community. (In the last eight years, for instance, OCLC has had only one price increase in its core products.)

By consistently operating in a prudent and businesslike manner as it pursues its public purposes, OCLC has been able to provide more than $1 billion in needed, high quality products and services for its members, and in doing so has helped libraries save millions of dollars. It is simultaneously able to take care of members' needs promptly, to take advantage of improvements in technology, and to undertake worthwhile *pro bono* projects for the benefit of libraries and their users. Financial independence has been a key element in enabling OCLC to make its public purposes a reality.

Membership Role in Governance

A third defining characteristic of OCLC is that it is a membership organization whose members have an important and institutionalized role in its governance. OCLC's governance structure has evolved since 1967 and has always been closely intertwined with the use of OCLC systems and products and the growth of the OCLC bibliographic database. The present governance structure, adopted in 1977, consists basically of General Members, the OCLC Users Council, and the OCLC Board of Trustees.

General members of OCLC are those libraries that do all their current cataloging online or via tapeload. General members elect delegates to three-year terms on the Users Council, with apportionment based on calculations of system use. The "delegate algorithm" which governs such apportionment is a closely watched and frequently debated topic.

The 60 elected delegates to Users Council bring a variety of perspectives and interests to OCLC. They come from many types and sizes of libraries and from varying positions within libraries. The Users Council meets for at least two full days three times a year. These meetings, which are attended by OCLC management and most members of the OCLC Board of Trustees, are not unlike traditional stockholders' meetings. Council delegates hear reports from OCLC management and outside experts, raise issues, exchange ideas, and pass resolutions. The sessions are routinely lively and informative as delegates take their "representative" functions very seriously. The Users Council not only plays a vital role in OCLC policy and planning, but also ratifies changes to OCLC's articles of incorporation and code of regulations and, perhaps most importantly, elects six members of the Board of Trustees.

Any discussion of Users Council must also include OCLC's 16 U.S. Regional Networks. From the beginning, when OCLC first introduced its products outside Ohio, independent regional networks have played a key role in bringing the benefits of OCLC participation to U.S. libraries. This partnership has been central to OCLC's growth and success in the past and will continue to be in the future. Each of these 16 independent networks has an agreement with OCLC to provide support, training and up-to-date information about OCLC products and services to their member libraries. Today, 99.9 percent of libraries in the U.S. participate in OCLC through a regional network. The networks have about 170 full-time staff who, in a typical year, train some 13,500 persons at over a thousand workshops and exhibit OCLC products at more than 200 conferences and user meetings. Network and OCLC User Support staff answer more than 24,000 support calls a year from libraries.

In addition to their front-line support role with libraries, regional networks are the vehicles for electing delegates to Users Council. They also nominate OCLC Product Advisory Committee members (OCLC has 17 advisory groups on products and services and programs that also meet on a regular basis), and advise OCLC directly through regular meetings of RONDAC (Regional OCLC Network Directors Advisory Committee).

The final say in OCLC's governance rests with its Board of Trustees. This 15-member Board is composed of six trustees elected by the Users Council (six-year terms); five trustees elected by the Board itself from fields outside librarianship such as law, finance, government, business, computer science, telecommunications, and marketing (four-year terms); and three board-elected trustees from the general library community (four-year terms). The President of OCLC is also an ex-officio trustee.

The Board of Trustees is responsible for setting strategic goals and policy, approving plans and programs for achieving those goals, hiring and firing the chief executive officer, approving annual budgets, overseeing audits and other reports pertaining to the basic financial condition of OCLC, and performing all of the traditional fiduciary and constituency duties related to such governing bodies. The four regular Board meetings each year last two days each and a fifth meeting, devoted to strategic planning, lasts three days. The time demands on OCLC Board members are demanding and continue to grow. And the Board's reputation for independence, involvement and willingness to deal directly with issues is well-known.

Clearly, the concept of membership governance influences all of OCLC's plans and decisions and is a major characteristic that distinguishes the OCLC-user relationship from the traditional vendor-customer one. Librarians at both large and small libraries have rightfully come to think of their institutions as stakeholders in OCLC with voices that require attention. This author believes strongly that OCLC members exert substantially greater power in the management and governance of OCLC than do the shareholders of publicly owned, for-profit organizations. OCLC's corporate democracy is real. In a meaningful sense, the President of OCLC faces the equivalent of an "annual shareholders' meeting" at least once a month.

The 25,000 libraries in 63 countries that participate in OCLC not only have an institutionalized voice and role in OCLC's governance, but they also deeply believe in library cooperation, in OCLC's broad public purposes, and in a constant dialogue on library-related issues. Indeed, the idealistic expectations of participating libraries often led Rowland Brown, OCLC's second president, to frequently say that: "OCLC is not a business, but a religion."[4]

OCLC TODAY

The OCLC the author has been privileged to lead for the last nine years is an international institution whose public purposes of furthering access to the world's information and reducing information costs are more vital than ever.

OCLC's campus has not only grown to 100 acres, it has also grown into a global force in scholarship, research and education. It is a busy place. Thousands of users, librarians and educators from all over the country visit each year to attend programs, training sessions, and meet with OCLC staff on a variety of matters. In 1994, more than 20,000 librarians participated in a two-hour OCLC videoconference on the electronic library at more than 750 downlink sites in North America and Europe. Thousands of people visit OCLC's Home Page on the World Wide Web each day. And hundreds of thousands of library users access OCLC's computer systems and services around the clock, around the world, 365 days a year.

Today, OCLC is one of the leading providers of computerized library services in the world. There are three main service areas: collections and technical services, resource sharing, and reference.

Collections and Technical Services

Collections and technical services in general and cataloging in particular remain at the heart of OCLC. While cataloging remains OCLC's principal source of revenue, its percentage of total net revenues has steadily declined from 72 percent in 1979 (the year that OCLC added the Interlibrary Loan system to its online offerings) to 36 percent in 1997. The OCLC Cataloging service handles over a billion online transactions annually, with message traffic running as high as 110 messages a second. Annually, libraries use OCLC to process some 40 million books and other materials via a spectrum of services that meet the needs of individual libraries' workflows and local systems.

Since the installation of a new, modular, high-performance $30-million cataloging and resource sharing system in 1992, OCLC has focused its activities in collections and technical services on enriching WorldCat, developing alternative methods for creating and delivering catalog records, improving productivity, and providing authority control services.

WorldCat now contains nearly 38 million records and over 660 million location listings. It spans over 4,000 years of recorded knowledge in 377 languages. It grows by two million original records a year, or 15 records a second. WorldCat is the most valuable asset that OCLC has, and one of the most valuable such assets in the world. And, OCLC works hard at maintaining the quality of this priceless resource. For example, OCLC continuously runs software that automatically updates and corrects subject and name authority records in WorldCat. OCLC member libraries, through the Enhance Program, also volunteer their expertise to correct and improve WorldCat records.

OCLC continuously seeks to enrich WorldCat through the addition of library collections from around the world, through both retrospective conversion and online cataloging. Recent major record conversion projects include Harvard University, the Consortium of University Research Libraries in the United Kingdom, the French Ministry of Education, Queensland University, University of Sao Paolo and Waseda University. OCLC has also recently loaded the Czech and Slovenian National Bibliographies into WorldCat. (Some 87 percent of the Czech records were original.)

Besides adding a steady stream of enhancements to its cataloging system throughout the 1990s, OCLC has also introduced new products and services that augment and complement online cataloging. OCLC PromptCat, for example, provides automated delivery of cataloging information with minimal staff intervention. In conjunction with PromptCat, OCLC has created the Cataloging In Publication Upgrade Program in which OCLC works with book vendors, publishers and the Library of Congress to accelerate the enhancement of CIP information in WorldCat. Some libraries have now outsourced portions of their cataloging to OCLC through the OCLC TechPro service. Most libraries, however, do their cataloging either online on OCLC or on their local systems. To make OCLC cataloging more accessible for local library systems, OCLC introduced Z39.50 access to WorldCat for cataloging. And to make budgeting for cataloging easier and simple, OCLC introduced subscription pricing for cataloging in 1997. Today, WorldCat is not only the most consulted reference database in higher education, it is also the most consulted bibliographic database for library cataloging departments around the world, with a hit rate of 94.6 percent for current materials.

As online public access catalogs have become the rule rather than the exception, libraries are finding that authority control adds precision and value to bibliographic information. In 1997, OCLC introduced its Authority Control Service, which provides software that lets libraries correct or modernize name, series, and subject headings in their catalogs.

Clearly, OCLC is now helping libraries get their cataloging records into their local systems and their materials out on their shelves faster than ever before. Moreover, as library materials flow through selection and ordering to cataloging and the bookshelf, their records are linked automatically to

WorldCat. This link is a crucial one, not only for technical services, but for public services such as resource sharing and reference.

Resource Sharing

If current ILL trends (8 million annually) continue, sometime in the year 2000, approximately 21 years after OCLC introduced the ILL system in 1979, some OCLC member library will conduct the 100 millionth online interlibrary loan. Over the last two decades, resource sharing, however, has become more than just interlibrary loan. In this vital area of library cooperation, OCLC has been working hard to provide a single integrated service for searching, interlibrary loan, and document delivery as well as to develop both mediated and non-mediated services for the library. (In this regard, it is interesting to note that three percent of interlibrary loans in research libraries in 1996 were initiated by library patrons via the OCLC FirstSearch service, a trend that is likely to grow rapidly.) The OCLC Union List enables libraries to inventory and monitor serials collections among self-defined groups of libraries, and it now supports 145 lists for 14,113 libraries. The OCLC ILL Fee Management service, introduced in 1996, is now processing more than 1,500 debit/credit interlibrary loan transactions a day, thus saving libraries from check-writing costs of between $30 and $75 apiece for such transactions. Thanks to ILL Fee Management, the Library of Congress was able to resume its international interlibrary loan service. The goal in all of the recent ILL enhancements, which include customized holdings, is to increase the productivity of the entire process.

OCLC SiteSearch software enables groups of libraries to now share resources not only more productively, but in exciting new ways. For example, the University System of Georgia uses OCLC software to deliver bibliographic, abstract, and full-text information to 34 academic libraries in Georgia through its GALILEO system. Faculty and students can use GALILEO to access library holdings, including journal articles, over the Word Wide Web whether they are in the library, their office, or their home. As Zell Miller, the Governor of Georgia, puts it: "GALILEO serves every one of our university system units with more resources than any of them could afford alone."

Reference Services

For its first 20 years, OCLC was by and large a computer library service for professional librarians, with services focused on cataloging and interlibrary loan. In the 1990s, however, OCLC has developed a series of new services designed for the end-users of information.

In 1991, OCLC introduced FirstSearch, which is designed specifically for use by the library patron. It is a new concept that provides the general public with online reference information that heretofore could only be obtained through a professional reference librarian. FirstSearch now provides users with bibliographic, abstract, and full-text information. Library users can now consult over 65 databases, including WorldCat, and look at catalog entries, abstracts of articles, and even order the full text of an article and get it either on their screen immediately or in paper form through the mail. FirstSearch requires no training. By 1997, FirstSearch ranked number one among online reference services in terms of connect time.

OCLC's approach to online reference service has been revolutionary. At the time of FirstSearch's introduction, one observer wrote:

> Libraries will be the real winners with FirstSearch because they will establish themselves as the foremost providers of online searching, rather than having to apologize for being unable to afford it. This comes at a perfect time, for the nation's libraries are under unprecedented pressure to justify their role. FirstSearch can help them demonstrate that they are indeed a uniquely valuable force in modern society, rather than archaic warehouses headed for extinction.[5]

OCLC has also been a pioneer in electronic publishing. In 1992, with the American Association for the Advancement of Science OCLC developed the world's first peer-reviewed, electronic, scholarly journal called the *Online Journal of Current Clinical Trials.* The journal was designed to get the results of clinical trials into the hands of medical practitioners six months faster than traditional print journals.

In June 1997, OCLC introduced the FirstSearch Electronic Collections Online service, which provides access to a large collection of academic journals, from many publishers, through a single Web interface that supports cross-journal searching and extensive browsing. FirstSearch Electronic Collections Online builds on more than a decade of research and development that OCLC has done in electronic journals and electronic publishing, including the now discontinued Guidon interface and Electronic Journals Online program. These pioneering efforts not only helped to set the stage for Electronic Collections Online, but also provided OCLC and member libraries with valuable and necessary real-world experience in electronic journals. Indeed, in a 1996 news release, the American Institute of Physics stated: "AIP and the remainder of the scientific and technical publishing community owe an enormous debt of gratitude to OCLC for its groundbreaking efforts in online journal publishing. OCLC made a high-risk, multimillion-dollar investment in the development of its EJO system and Guidon client, at a time when the World Wide Web was yet to be invented. Clearly, their efforts have advanced the development of online journals at a much faster pace than would otherwise have been the case."

In addition to collections and technical services, resource sharing, and reference, OCLC is active in other selected areas as well. Preservation Resources, an OCLC division based in Bethlehem, Pennsylvania, provides a full range of preservation services for libraries and archives–superior microfilming of materials, editorial preparation, storage, access, digital scanning, and distribution. OCLC Forest Press publishes the Dewey Decimal Classification, now in its 21st edition, and also offers an electronic version of what is the world's most widely used classification system. And, at this writing, OCLC was starting to deploy a new, TCP/IP telecommunications network that will provide libraries with more reliable, high-quality telecommunications with OCLC via the Internet and World Wide Web at dramatically lower cost.

The OCLC of today is also a global organization. OCLC now serves over 2,280 libraries in 62 countries outside the U.S. International activities now account for almost ten percent of OCLC's revenues, which in 1997 translated into some $13 million. OCLC serves these libraries through four divisions–OCLC Asia Pacific, OCLC Canada, OCLC Europe, OCLC Latin America and the Caribbean. Since 1996, OCLC has also operated a service center at Tsinghua University in Beijing. At this writing, OCLC had major new projects under way in Australia, Brazil, Germany, Israel, Malaysia, Mexico, New Zealand, Poland and South Africa.

The OCLC of today is also a major research organization. The OCLC Office of Research, established in 1978, is one of the world's leading centers devoted to the problems and challenges for libraries in the Information Age. OCLC spends about $5 million a year on basic research, much more on applied research. Over the years, the OCLC membership has reaped enormous benefits from this effort. A few of the new products and services introduced in the last five years that got started in the OCLC Office of Research include: FirstSearch, SiteSearch, FirstSearch Electronic Collections Online, Guidon, WebZ, PromptCat, PURLS, NetFirst and Authorities software. These innovations are helping libraries not only cope with the present but build for the future. They grew out of a sustained research and development effort coupled with an ongoing strategic planning process at OCLC that focuses on library needs. The Office of

Research gives OCLC and its member libraries an infrastructure and an ongoing, systematic, interactive process for dealing with rapidly changing technology in the emerging digital, global community.

To sum up, the OCLC of today provides integrated solutions for libraries at key points in the flow of information from publisher to library to end user. Libraries can use OCLC products and services to build and operate a global digital library that provides seamless access to both print and electronic information for library users when and where they need it, at a price they can afford. Equally important, this digital library can now be customized to meet local needs and concerns. These integrated solutions, coupled with a global perspective and a strong commitment to library research, make OCLC an important international library resource.

OCLC TOMORROW

Former OCLC Board Chair Edward G. Holley was fond of saying that OCLC "has more opportunities on its plate than it can say grace over." Indeed, choosing from among a plate full of opportunities is the principal blessing and challenge for the OCLC of tomorrow. In the 1990s, OCLC has been employing an ongoing strategic planning process to regularly identify and pursue the choices that best serve the OCLC membership and mission.

In 1991, OCLC sent to member libraries a summary of the first OCLC strategic plan, "Journey to the 21st Century," which said in essence that in the 1990 to 1995 time frame, OCLC would install a new telecommunications network, install a new online system for cataloging and resource sharing and launch a new core business in reference services.

By 1993, OCLC was running ahead of schedule and had already accomplished the initial goals set forth in the plan. The OCLC Board of Trustees then articulated three new strategic priorities for OCLC–growing a new online reference service, enhancing the cataloging and resource sharing system, and expanding internationally.

By 1996, much of the original 1991 OCLC strategic plan and the Board's additions had become outdated, not because the ideas were wrong, but because OCLC had done what it had set out to do.

The new OCLC strategic plan, published in September 1997, is called "Beyond 2000" and builds on the 1991 document, sets new directions and refocuses strategic priorities. This updated plan is the result of a year-long process that involved consulting with and listening to all of OCLC's major constituencies–the Board of Trustees, Users Council, U.S. regional networks, business partners, international distributors, advisory groups and many individual libraries and users. It should be noted that throughout this planning process, OCLC's overall vision has remained the same–to provide seamless access to bibliographic, abstract and full-text information when and where people need it, in the form they want, and at a price they can afford.

In brief, OCLC's strategy over the next decade will be to pursue four major goals. The first goal is to integrate and enhance all OCLC core services by providing easy and seamless access to information. The second is to innovate by providing new, cost-effective, electronic alternatives such as electronic archiving and new telecommunications technologies. The third is to internationalize by increasing global expansion and perspective. And, the fourth goal is to inform by adding educational services for the library and education communities, which OCLC is already doing with the OCLC Institute, which was established in early 1997.

As OCLC pursues its new goals, however, there are some important fundamentals that will not change. OCLC will continue to be a nonprofit, membership, library organization. It will continue to focus on pursuing its public purposes of furthering access to the world's information and reducing information costs. It will continue to be characterized by maintaining financial independence and active membership participation in governance. It will continue to rely primarily on its regional networks for marketing, support and training for products and services in the U.S. Outside the U.S., OCLC will continue to seek appropriate partnerships and alliances in individual countries and to work within the culture of individual countries. While understanding and taking full advantage of the value of technological change, OCLC will also continue to emphasize the enduring, old-fashioned, non-technical values–cooperation, collaboration, resource sharing, democratizing access to information. Finally, OCLC will continue to emphasize quality, service, and doing a few things exceptionally well.

Taken together, these tangible and intangible fundamentals constitute a formula for success that ties innovation to tradition, tools to people, and individual libraries to a library commons. It is a formula that has enabled OCLC to contribute significantly to the library community and to the public good for thirty years. If it continues to be followed, it is the author's firm belief that for OCLC and libraries and library users, the best still lies ahead.

NOTES

1. Hall, Peter Dobkin. 1978. "A Historical Overview of the Private Nonprofit Sector," in *The Nonprofit Sector,* ed. Walter W. Powell: 3. New Haven and London: Yale University Press.

2. Ohio College Library Center. 1968. *Annual Report 1967/68*. Columbus: Ohio College Library Center: 4.

3. OCLC Online Computer Library Center. 1992. *Annual Report 1991/92*. Dublin, Ohio: OCLC Online Computer Library Center: 23.

4. Frederick G. Kilgour, OCLC's founder, first executive director, and first president, served as president and chief executive officer from 1967 to 1980. Rowland C. W. Brown served as OCLC's second president and chief executive officer from 1980 to 1989. K. Wayne Smith, the current president and CEO, joined OCLC in January 1989.

5. O'Leary, Mick. 1992. "FirstSearch Takes the Lead." *Information Today* (February): 11-13.

APPENDIX

OCLC: Thirty Years of Technological Innovation

1967
OCLC Articles of Incorporation signed

1968
MARC II format created at Library of Congress

1969
First LC-MARC II Distribution Service tape, containing approximately 1,000 records, issued

OCLC offline catalog card production starts

1970
Xerox Sigma 5 computer installed at OCLC for online system

1971
August 26, 1971–online shared cataloging system begins operation

October 18, 1971–online system starts accepting member input cataloging

1972
3 Networks join OCLC:
  CCLC
  NELINET
  PRLC

Standards for Input Cataloging issued

OCLC control number access

1973
M100 Terminal Introduced (Beehive)

Extended search function is activated–users may now retrieve and view up
to 256 database entries under a specific search key

1974
Dial-access

4 Networks join OCLC:
FAUL
FEDLINK
AMIGOS
PALINET

CONSER (Cooperative ONline SERials) program begins building database of authoritative serials records (500,000 by 1991)

WorldCat totals one million bibliographic records

1975
XEROX Sigma 9

First Sigma 9 is installed on Online System

4 Networks join OCLC:
MLNC
ILLINET
SOLINET
SUNY

1976
5 Networks join OCLC:
BCR
CAPCON
INCOLSA
MLC
WILS

Western Service Center (PACNET) established

Implementation of card production for MARC II formats in addition to Books

Corporate name index added to online system

ALL PRODUCE function

Government Printing Office starts producing Monthly Catalog of Government Publications from OCLC-MARC tapes

1977
4 Networks join OCLC:
PACNET
MINITEX
NEBASE
MRLN

1978
OHIONET established

OCLC Users Council meets for first time

Office of Research formed

M105 Terminal introduced

1979
Interlibrary Loan Subsystem introduced

Canadian library is first international participant

OCLC libraries in all 50 states

1980
Online Name-Address Directory activated

OCLC bibliographic database converted to AACR2 form

Online retrieval by Government Document number is added

Serials Union List

Holdings display alphabetically by state or region

1981
Acquisitions Subsystem

OCLC Europe formed

1982
University of Minnesota becomes first tapeloader

Linked Systems Project (LSP) begins

1983
United States Newspaper Program

Merge Holdings

Merge Holdings capability is activated

LS/2000 system launched

ILL Subsystem is linked to Name-Address Directory

WorldCat totals 10 million bibliographic records

1984
Major Microforms

Uninterruptible Power System (UPS) installed for Online System

M300 Workstation introduced

Interlibrary Loan MicroEnhancer available

Enhance Program

1985
MICROCON introduced

1986
2nd AACR2 conversion of the database

TAPECON and Group Access Capability (GAC)

1987
CJK350 system for cataloging Chinese, Japanese, and Korean materials introduced

Online access to LC subject authority records

Search CD450 introduced

1988
OCLC Forest Press publishes 20th edition of the Dewey Decimal Classification

CAT CD450 introduced

OCLC/AMIGOS Collection Analysis Systems Available

1989
Graph-Text patent

M386/16 Workstation introduced

1990
The American Association for the Advancement of Science (AAAS) and OCLC begin a joint electronic publishing venture

EPIC Service introduced

New technological platform for cataloging and resource sharing (PRISM service)

GOVDOC service introduced

1991
FirstSearch introduced

M386sx Workstation introduced

New X.25 telecommunications network installed

1992

Online Journal of Current Clinical Trials, world's first peer-reviewed electronic medical journal, introduced

Preservation Resources receives patent for preservation camera exposure system

Migration to new OCLC cataloging and resource-sharing system completed

1993

Keyword searching

ILL link to FirstSearch

Sunday hours for OCLC Cataloging and Resource Sharing service

Automated authority corrections software applied to WorldCat

Automated tape management system installed

M486DXI Workstation introduced

Electronic Dewey introduced

Telecommunications Linking Program (TLP)

1994

OCLC SiteSearch software introduced

29 million records in WorldCat

Electronic Journals Online program

Gateway software for local systems interface to OCLC

Name-Address Directory, Union List and CJK Plus up on new technological platform

Internet Cataloging Project

OCLC ILL Transfer

E-mail submission of WorldCat error corrections

1995

Authorities capabilities

PromptCat introduced

Internet access to OCLC cataloging and resource sharing

ILL Fee Management

OCLC WebZ Server

Preservation Resources scanning/indexing service

Harvard Resource File

ILL Custom Holdings

NetFirst database of Internet resources

1996

MARC Format integration completed

OCLC Authority Control service introduced

OCLC CatCD for Windows

Custom Holdings for Union List

World Wide Web access to FirstSearch

NetFirst database

21st edition of Dewey Decimal Classification published

1997

OCLC ILL Micro Enhancer for Windows software

Electronic archiving projects in seven libraries

FirstSearch Electronic Collections Online introduced

TCP/IP telecommunciations network installation starts

Index

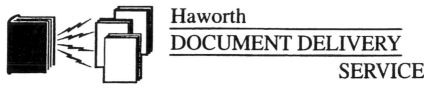

Haworth
DOCUMENT DELIVERY
SERVICE

This valuable service provides a single-article order form for any article from a Haworth journal.

- *Time Saving:* No running around from library to library to find a specific article.
- *Cost Effective:* All costs are kept down to a minimum.
- *Fast Delivery:* Choose from several options, including same-day FAX.
- *No Copyright Hassles:* You will be supplied by the original publisher.
- *Easy Payment:* Choose from several easy payment methods.

Open Accounts Welcome for...
- Library Interlibrary Loan Departments
- Library Network/Consortia Wishing to Provide Single-Article Services
- Indexing/Abstracting Services with Single Article Provision Services
- Document Provision Brokers and Freelance Information Service Providers

---

MAIL or *FAX* THIS ENTIRE ORDER FORM TO:

Haworth Document Delivery Service
The Haworth Press, Inc.
10 Alice Street
Binghamton, NY 13904-1580

or FAX: 1-800-895-0582
or CALL: 1-800-342-9678
9am-5pm EST

PLEASE SEND ME PHOTOCOPIES OF THE FOLLOWING SINGLE ARTICLES:

1) Journal Title: _____
   Vol/Issue/Year: _____ Starting & Ending Pages: _____
   Article Title: _____
   _____

2) Journal Title: _____
   Vol/Issue/Year: _____ Starting & Ending Pages: _____
   Article Title: _____
   _____

3) Journal Title: _____
   Vol/Issue/Year: _____ Starting & Ending Pages: _____
   Article Title: _____
   _____

4) Journal Title: _____
   Vol/Issue/Year: _____ Starting & Ending Pages: _____
   Article Title: _____
   _____

(See other side for Costs and Payment Information)

COSTS: Please figure your cost to order quality copies of an article.

1. Set-up charge per article: $8.00

   ($8.00 × number of separate articles) _____

2. Photocopying charge for each article:

   1-10 pages: $1.00 _____

   11-19 pages: $3.00 _____

   20-29 pages: $5.00 _____

   30+ pages: $2.00/10 pages _____

3. Flexicover (optional): $2.00/article _____

4. Postage & Handling: US: $1.00 for the first article/

   $.50 each additional article _____

   Federal Express: $25.00 _____

   Outside US: $2.00 for first article/

   $.50 each additional article_____

5. Same-day FAX service: $.35 per page _____

   GRAND TOTAL: _____

METHOD OF PAYMENT: (please check one)

❏ Check enclosed   ❏ Please ship and bill. PO # _____
   (sorry we can ship and bill to bookstores only! All others must pre-pay)

❏ Charge to my credit card: ❏ Visa; ❏ MasterCard; ❏ Discover;
   ❏ American Express;

Account Number:_____ Expiration date:_____

Signature: *X*_____

Name: _____ Institution: _____

Address: _____

_____

City: _____ State:_____ Zip:_____

Phone Number: _____ FAX Number: _____

MAIL or *FAX* THIS ENTIRE ORDER FORM TO:

Haworth Document Delivery Service | **or FAX:** 1-800-895-0582
The Haworth Press, Inc. | **or CALL:** 1-800-342-9678
10 Alice Street | 9am-5pm EST)
Binghamton, NY 13904-1580 |